Health Awakening Series, Book

The Postpartum Recovery Program™

How to Rejuvenate your Hormones, Body, & Mind After Childbirth

by Dr. Lia G. Andrews, DAOM, L.Ac.

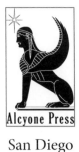

Alcyone Press

San Diego

Published by Alcyone Press
San Diego, CA
www.AlcyonePress.com

ISBN-10: 0989326039
ISBN-13: 978-0-9893260-3-2

Library of Congress Control Number: 2014908431

This book is intended to be informational and should not be considered a substitute for advice from a medical professional, whom the reader should consult before beginning any diet or exercise regimen, and before taking any dietary supplements or other medications. The author and publisher expressly disclaim responsibility for any adverse effects arising from the use or application of the information in this book.

For more information please see www.PostpartumRecoveryProgram.com

For information on Dr. Andrews' clinic in San Diego, please see www.CinnabarAcupuncture.com

For rights and permission inquiries please contact the author through her website: www.LiaAndrews.com

Health Awakening Series:
Book 1: 7 Times a Woman; Ancient Wisdom on Health & Beauty for Every Stage of Your Life
Book 2: The Postpartum Recovery Program™; How to Rejuvenate your Hormones, Body, & Mind After Childbirth

Editors: Lia Andrews, Judith Andrews, Jacquie Lowell, Anita Edmonson
Layout Design & Graphic Editing: PXPDesign.com
Cover Design: Lia Andrews
Author Photograph: Judith Andrews
Illustrations: Lia Andrews

Dedication

To the Divine Mother

and

To my grandfather, Dr. João Rodrigues Goulart (vovô),

who delivered countless babies and honored women before it was trendy.

Contents

Acknowledgements

I want to thank all the many people, whose contributions have made this book possible.

I want to thank Miya Uchida of PXP Design for being a dear friend and teacher. She designed the inside of this book. She patiently tutored me in InDesign and Illustrator. Her ingenuity, work ethic, and attention to detail were necessary for the creation of this book.

Thank you, Dr. Judith Andrews, for organizing our notes, expediting the process of writing this book.

Thank you to Dr. Jiang Zheng who gave me a copy of Dr. Shuqi Zhuang's book on postpartum care for me to translate while I was in my doctoral program, which was the basis for my capstone, and eventually inspired this book. Dr. Lily Chang was so generous in her time and talent to verify my translation.

Thank you to Judith Andrews, Anita Edmonson, Jacquie Lowell, and Robyn Caringella for editing and giving feedback.

I want to thank my mom, Dr. Judith Andrews, for her constant support and technical insights. A big thank you to my teachers who influenced my practice in unique ways. I want to thank my human, plant, and animal friends, my family, and my patients and for the divine guidance I have received.

Forward: That's Normal, Right?

by Dr. Veronica Anover, Ph.D.

I am the mother of the most gorgeous and sweet boy. Of course I think he is the sweetest and the greatest, I am his mom! That's normal, right?

Like so many women, I carefully planned my pregnancy. I made sure that my husband of 11 years (at the time) and I held steady jobs, that we were responsible enough to bring a new life into this world, and that our health was at its peak. I was 34 years old when I became pregnant. The second I found out that I was expecting, I was the happiest woman on earth! I had conceived a baby with the love of my life. That's normal, right?

I made an appointment with an OBGYN near my residence (I was new to the area, therefore I did not have a network of doctors yet) and I was a little disappointed when the doctor could not see me right away. I had to wait six weeks before that first doctor's visit. I understood later that it is a cautionary measure in case I miscarried. The day of my visit I was jubilant. I was going to find out more about that little bean growing in my womb, and more importantly I was going to be reassured that everything was going well. I surrounded myself with books about expectant parents in English, in French and in Spanish that I ordered from local bookstores, France and Spain. (I am a native of France). I avidly read the first few chapters and got more and more excited – and at times more and more worried, knowing the risks that could arise- as I read along. That's normal, right?

None of my books warned me that on that first visit I was going to have a vaginal ultrasound. I went to the doctor's office thinking that I was going to receive a "belly" ultrasound. You know the one where the technician applies a thick layer of gel on your belly and moves in circles, right and left, with a magic wand that is connected to a computer screen where you may see your munchkin for the first time? Well, to my dismay, that ended up not being the case. I felt somewhat violated (like when a thief enters your bedroom and opens all the drawers in search of a hidden booty) although I had been told seconds before the "break in" about this initial test. When I asked the doctor why she had chosen to use this method she sharply answered: "We must discard that you are carrying twins, or even triplets; at your age, it is not uncommon." Oh, ok, I thought. I guess I am an older mom and as such I could have used medication to produce more ovules during ovulation. Ok, makes sense, right? (Mind you, she never asked me if I had used such medication!)

To make a long story short, I ditched that doctor after my second appointment when she tried to convince me that I had a blood type that was not mine! "You are O positive," she said. "No, I know I am A positive; my entire family has that blood type, and when I had surgery many years ago, that is what the doctors told me I was." "That is impossible," the "mean" doctor replied (by now, she was very upset with me for contradicting her). Since she never considered a lab error and she kept on insisting that I had a wrong blood type, I decided to never, ever come back and to switch doctors and even clinics. I was proud to have taken action and not to have doubted of myself.

The second doctor I found was highly recommended and she turned out to be a gem. She was very sweet and knowledgeable; very professional as well. She was part of a group of OBGYNs and I knew that any of her partners could be on call the day I would deliver. As a matter of fact, the office scheduled follow up appointments with each doctor at the end of my third trimester so that I could meet all of them. Of course I was crossing my fingers so that my doctor, the one I trusted and knew the most about my baby and me, would be delivering my bundle of joy. That's normal, right?

I have nothing major to report about my pregnancy except that my French and Spanish books recommended a maximum weight gain of 10-12 kilos (22-26 pounds) and my US ones 30 pounds. Being the good student I have always been, I gained a total of 28 pounds. (Nice compromise!) Of course, the day I felt my little soccer-player-to-be kicking my belly and making somersaults, tears of joy and immense love rolled uncontrollably on my cheeks. Tears of relief as well. My little guy is alive and kicking! (Pun intended!)

There are many differences between American and French pre-natal and post-natal care. I will spare you here issues about nutrition, exercise, lactation, body care and recovery, etc. Instead I will share with you my delivery and my post-delivery experience, which are at the heart of my story.

In preparation for the arrival of our baby, my husband and I eagerly attended the prenatal classes that were offered through the clinic and met other expecting parents who were following and practicing the breathing exercises faithfully and methodically. (Also called the Lamaze exercises, named after a French obstetrician, Dr. Fernand Lamaze from the 1940s).

Well, the big day arrived and at 2:00 a.m. when my first contractions started on a Thursday at the beginning of August. We left the house calmly but without wasting a single minute, and we signed in the front desk at the clinic half an hour later. I was quickly admitted and placed in a beautiful room that looked more like a cozy bedroom than a hospital one. I got hooked to a monitor that showed the baby's heartbeat. I was beyond feeling excitement and anticipation, ready as can be to welcome my little guy, hold him and kiss him and look at him with all my love. And that is normal too, right?

At 10:00 a.m. (more than 6 hours after been admitted) since I was not dilating fast enough and still having contractions more and more painful each time, the doctor on call (big misfortune, it was not "MY" doctor, but one of her colleagues) broke my water and gave me medication to expedite the process. By that time, after trying the hot shower, the walking down the hallway and the squeezing to death my poor hubby's hand, my contractions were so painful that I begged for some relief. The anesthesiologist injected the epidural on my spine and I became temporarily paraplegic but pain free! I will figure out how to push later, I thought. Later came much, much later and finally at 9:40 p.m. my baby boy was born. He was healthy and he was here. That is all that mattered for now. At some point during my delivery, between "push-breath-push-breath," I saw the doctor approaching with big scissors and blood splattered all over the white wall in front of me. It was strange not to have felt a thing even though I knew that the blood was undeniably mine from an episiotomy. But who cares, the doctor is doing her best, and my baby cannot suffer as he comes through. I must have been pushing for hours (it is a blur and details escape from my memory) when I heard the doctor say in a very smooth and confident voice: "if the baby does not come out at the next push, after I use the suction cup, we are going to have to do a C-section." "Hell no!" I thought, "No way. After all this pushing, my baby is coming this way!"

And he did, and it was the most amazing feeling I have ever felt in my life, when I first saw my little guy with his big blue eyes looking intensely at me as if he were checking me out. "Hmm…, so this is who my mom is! Cool, not too bad! She seems tired, but nice!" The most incredible feeling and boost of love I have ever experienced was when my husband (who had not left my side for a second during these long hours) took our baby boy in his big arms, and his hands were bigger than our little son's head. I could cry again, just evoking these unique, intense, tender and loving moments. That's normal, right?

Meanwhile, the doctor was stitching me up to repair the damage left by the incision after she cut me wide open "down there" with the scissors (or what seemed to be scissors.)

The next morning, the pain "down there" was excruciating but I figured, "it is normal", right? Someone came to show me briefly, very briefly, how to breastfeed my baby and after two days I was sent home with my newborn and his new dad. And that is when I lost myself. That is when I became alienated with my Self, with a big "S". Who am I? What have I done? I cannot do this, this is too hard, I am an awful mom, and I am in deep, deep pain still, 6 weeks after the arrival of my little one. I shared these thoughts with my doctor (the OBGYN who had given me my prenatal care) and I shared my pain with her too. I was told that everything was normal. OK, so if it is normal, I just need to suck it up, right?

Except that after two years (yes, two years), I was still in pain "down South" and I was barely starting to get acquainted with myself again. I could not recognize my changed body with its stubborn excess weight, my hemorrhoids not forgiving me for all that pushing, and my sensitive breasts from the lactation. I never ceased to go back to my doctor, but each time I saw a different one from her group and all coincided on the same verdict: I was healing beautifully and the way I felt was due to lack of sleep. So, I assumed that was normal, right? The best was what one of the doctors told me about my pain: "Have another baby and it will feel better." Really? You repair a tear with another tear. Normal. If you have pain in your vaginal area caused by a delivery, you must have another baby so that you will tear again and hopefully the second time around, the stitches will be better placed, or better done. I see.

But that did not do it for me and I started to lose my patience. I happened to go to Europe that summer, and I made an appointment with my gynecologist, an older man who had been around for a while and who had seen and performed many deliveries. It only took one glance for him to assess the situation. I had a very thick scar tissue that had formed with many different layers. I was only staying a few weeks in Europe and surgery while on vacation was not an option.

I came back to the States and requested an appointment with "MY" OBGYN. The one I trusted who knew me best. I explained the situation to her, told her about her colleagues dismissing my issues and how fed up I was. I demanded that something be done to fix my problem that one of her colleagues had caused. She "observed the scene" and concluded that indeed something needed to be done. I was going to have reparative surgery, or as I like to call it, plastic surgery! I will end up with a brand new "me" inside. My doctor explained how she was going to perform the surgery and I decided it was a go. My "plastic" surgery was a success even though the doctor had never performed any surgery like this one before. After my surgery, I expressed my gratitude to my doctor for addressing and fixing my problem and I told her that I could not go back to her clinic. Her colleagues clearly demonstrated a lack of professionalism by ignoring my pain complaints and by trying to convince me that I was "healing beautifully".

It helps that I am educated (I have a Ph.D.) and that I became my own health advocate. I wish I had lost patience earlier. Two years is a lot. However I am glad that I demanded my problem be fixed as I felt in my right. I did not buy the "healing beautifully" although it took me a few years to realize that things were not going to get better with time. I urge you to question your doctors when you have doubts and to demand care when you need it. Trust your gut and do not stay with a doctor who does not listen to your concerns.

Because it is not normal to have pain past six weeks after you have delivered a baby –without complications-, and certainly it is not normal to have pain for two years after your delivery; it is not normal to have to resolve to a second tear in order to fix your first tear; it is not normal to feel like being a mom is insurmountable; and it is not normal to be dismissed by doctors.

What is normal is to be in pain for several weeks, to have the "baby blues" (and to be treated for it, although not all women have them), to be told how to recover your body (so that later on you do not have complications with incontinence, for example) and to be told the truth even if it means admitting that your procedure needs to be fixed.

Dr. Veronica Anover, Ph.D. is a Professor in the Modern Language Studies Department and a Global Studies Program affiliate. She developed and started the French Minor and the French Club at California State University San Marcos. She has developed courses for the French and Spanish Programs as well as Global Studies, such as her new course on Spanish for the Medical Field. Dr. Anover was department Chair from Fall 2006 until Fall 2009. In addition she served as Coordinator and Supervisor of the Spanish Graduate Teaching Assistants. As such she offered workshops on methodology and pedagogy, she conducted classroom observations and she held regular meetings with the GTAs to discuss best teaching practices. Her fields of expertise are Second Language Acquisition and contemporary French and Spanish women writers. She is particularly interested on the subjects of motherhood, mother-daughter relationships and pluriculturalism. She has co-authored several French and Spanish textbooks from beginner to intermediate levels. She is also a collaborator in the French Review where she regularly publishes. Dr. Anover is passionate about teaching and she has been the recipient of several teaching awards.

Introduction

This book translates the Chinese and Taiwanese postpartum tradition into a program that Western women can follow. These are powerful practices that literally transform the health of women after childbirth. American women in particular are not supported during the postpartum month. Through my masters and doctoral studies, and practicing in my own clinic, I observed how many women went into their postpartum unaware of what to expect and how to handle it, and thus devastated their health. It was a sad and unnecessary occurrence.

I was introduced to *zuò yuè zi* (坐月子), or Chinese postpartum recovery, by my TCM gynecology teacher Dr. Shaoting Jing during my master's program. It was not widely taught in acupuncture schools so I felt privileged that she thought to share that information with us. Later during my doctoral program I received another nudge when my gynecology teacher Dr. Jiang Zhang mailed me a copy of Dr. Shuqi Zhuang's book on Taiwanese postpartum care[1] to translate for my doctoral capstone.[2] Over the years I pieced together information from various sources. Through clinical experiences I learned to adapt dietary recommendations and practices to my patients.

In order for you to understand why I am so passionate about balancing women's health at key times in their lives, you need to know my story....

It was past 11pm when we finally got to our seats on the plane departing Rio de Janeiro for Miami. It had been a long day. My Brazilian grandfather had held on during our visit, but today, knowing we were leaving, his health had taken a turn for the worse. A former physician, he had been a staunch lifelong atheist following an unfortunate period spent at an austere boarding school run by German Protestants, complete with cold baths on winter mornings. In the last few weeks, however, he would comment to us on the deceased relatives who had come to visit him, and today he seemed to drift between this world and the next.

My mom made one last call to her parent's house as my father took my brother and I on the plane. My grandmother said they were taking my grandfather to the ER. Just as we were being seated, my mom came on to tell us what was happening. She told us to go home to North Carolina and that she would stay with her family. I wanted to stay too. For myself, I wish I had, but for my younger brother I am glad I did not.

Her leaving prompted airline security to be suspicious and it was a minor commotion for her to be let back out. I felt an emptiness as the airplane sped down the runway and I watched the *Cidade Maravilhosa*,[3] alight in her full majesty, falling away as we took flight.

---

1. Shuqi Zhuang. *Postpartum Recovery Program; a Manual of Rules and Recipes for the Postpartum Woman.* (Taiwan: Guang He Chu Ban She, 2005). ISBN 9578807015

2. Andrews, Lia. "Partial Translation of 'Postpartum Recovery Program; a Manual of Rules and Recipes for the Postpartum Woman.'" (DAOM capstone, Pacific College of Oriental Medicine, 2013). Available for free download here: www.academia.edu/4778907/PARTIAL_TRANSLATION_OF_POSTPARTUM_RECOVERY_PROGRAM_A_MANUAL_OF_RULES_AND_RECIPES_FOR_THE_POSTPARTUM_WOMAN

3. "Marvelous City" in Portuguese, a title bequeathed to the city of Rio by writer, composer André Filho.

I do not remember much of what happened after we arrived in the U.S. Before we knew it, my brother and I were being driven to upstate New York to stay with my paternal grandparents until my mom returned, so that my father could devote himself to his work. As we all waved him goodbye, my grandparents, my brother, and I stood together as strangers.

My brother and I were on our own. We would leave the house at sunrise each day and return when the street lights came on. We enjoyed new freedoms, friendships, and adventures and even faced off with roaming local bullies.

It was amidst all of this that, at 11 ½ years old, I got my first period. I did not tell anyone. I knew what it was and there was no one to tell. Luckily, I bled very little and was able to get by with tissue paper. It was only about a month later when my mom came to get us that I told her. I remember her being very sad about this. When she got her first period her father had thrown her a party and invited the whole family. It had been a big celebration into womanhood.

After my period came, my once vibrant health began to change. My periods were wildly irregular, though my mom thought this was normal in the beginning. However, the irregularity never stopped. Sometimes it would be 6 months, sometimes 2 weeks. And the periods themselves could be light and almost imperceptible or else heavy and incapacitating. I also developed severe acne, joint pain, and mysterious headaches. Doctors offered little in the way of understanding or solutions. I started to feel hopeless and depressed about my condition, which prompted one doctor to recommend Prozac, to which I did not respond well. Out of desperation my mom took me at age 15 to see a naturopathic physician who suspected a pituitary tumor, which a subsequent MRI confirmed. Conventional care offered risky laser surgery, so my mom took me to see an acupuncturist.

On that first visit I had a vision and experienced a paradigm shift. Over the next few months I began to make connections between what I ate, did, and thought and how my body felt. My periods started becoming regular. One year later an MRI showed no tumor present.

This experience deeply influenced both my mom and me. I was pre-med in college, but began to realize that it was not through allopathic medicine that I would help people. Upon graduation, my mom and I enrolled in acupuncture school together.

Our education in Traditional Chinese Medicine (TCM)[4] involved years of learning and continuous personal healing. It was during this time that I became focused on the significance of women's cycles as I observed the patterns emerging of early menstrual imbalances, fertility and postpartum issues, and menopausal symptoms in my patients. The hormonal turmoil I experienced as a pre-teen was my first awakening. It showed me in my own body how important it is to keep the physical body balanced as a foundation for happiness and spiritual growth. It also brought me to TCM which gave me the tools to understand these connections.

---

4. There is some discussion on what to call the traditional medicine of China, which has disseminated throughout Asia, and more recently the world. TCM is the most common term but is limiting. Other terms include Traditional Asian Medicine, Traditional Oriental Medicine, and simply Chinese medicine. These terms encompass a complex philosophy of disease pattern diagnosis, treatment strategy, acupuncture, herbology, qigong and tai chi, diet therapy, cupping, massage, gua sha, and structural adjustments.

It was after we had run our clinic, Cinnabar Acupuncture, for 5 years and I had finished my doctorate. Already overworked, I was overtaken by the need to write. Ten years of clinical experience have now made three things clear:

1) Healing women's cycles is critical for women's health, and most women are unaware of this.

2) Although the details of each woman's case are different, there is a collective story that wants to be told.

3) There is a change happening on the planet that cannot occur without empowered women, and the only way women can feel truly empowered is when we understand and honor our womanhood.

We must embrace fully our first menstruation (and everyone thereafter), our pregnancies (if that is our choice), our postpartum, and our second spring (menopause).

Society does not support this honoring. Decades after the feminist revolution we are still being told ever so subtly that to succeed in the world; to be seen and honored, we must stuff our womanliness to stand in the company of men, just as I had at 11 years old stuffed tissue paper in my panties and carried on. We are told to not run or throw, or react in various situations "like a girl," implying that there is something wrong with the way we females naturally do things.

As grown women we are fed advertising promising to mask or stop our periods so we can get back to doing things like normal. After all "who says" you need to get your period every month? Apparently we also need endless deodorizing products to keep away the stench "down there", while there don't seem to be any such products for men. Then there is the unspeakable horror of what lies ahead. After women have babies or approach menopause, they lose their beauty, the only power that their femininity affords.

What if none of this is really true? What if our collective suffering has come not from being born women, but from the extent to which we accept these myths about womanhood instead of learning how our bodies work, and claiming our female power?

I was fortunate enough to have a mom raised to love her womanliness. Not as some cultural caricature of high heels or a demure affect, but as a process of growing to know and embrace her whole self, her true self, and to share her gifts with the world.

I was fortunate again to find a form of medicine that could explain the workings of women in detail. Our cycles are here to keep us connected with ourselves and with the world around us in a way that is more difficult for men, because their cycles are less obvious. My intention is to convince you that your womanhood, cycles and all, is a gift.

In the next chapters I will show how ancient Chinese concepts and modern Western developments can afford modern women the best of both worlds. The Postpartum Recovery Program™ will empower you during your birthing and postpartum period. It will transform what can be a drain on your health and wellbeing into an opportunity to improve your health, even beyond how it was before you were pregnant.

Guide to Reading this Book

Attempts were made to accommodate a wider audience of patients, practitioners in other health fields, and the general public. The first three chapters in the beginning of the book and glossary of terminology in the appendix section seek to educate laypeople on the fundamentals of this medicine. Parentheses and footnotes are included throughout to clarify technical or historical significance.

Chinese herbs are listed in Mandarin pin yin followed by the common English name in parentheses. Appendix A at the end of the book lists the herbs with their pharmaceutical and botanical names as well. The Resources section guides you where to find them. Traditional Chinese Medical terms are capitalized to make them visually distinct. Common words are capitalized when they are used in a Traditional Chinese Medical context. For example, "Spleen" is capitalized when referring to the organ system in charge of transforming and transporting food, etc. If the biological functioning of the spleen organ was intended, then "spleen" would be in lower case.

I want to clarify the term Traditional Chinese Medicine (TCM) as used in this book. TCM is often used to describe only the standardized traditional medicine of China created by post-revolutionary China and devoid of all local variations and possible destabilizing concepts. My exposure to the traditional medicine of China is broader. I went to a lineage-based Daoist school and learned from teachers with varied backgrounds. I also include in this book Taiwanese traditions that were not influenced by post-revolutionary mainland China. I choose to use the term TCM to include all the traditional Chinese medical practices and modern global evolution of this medicine.

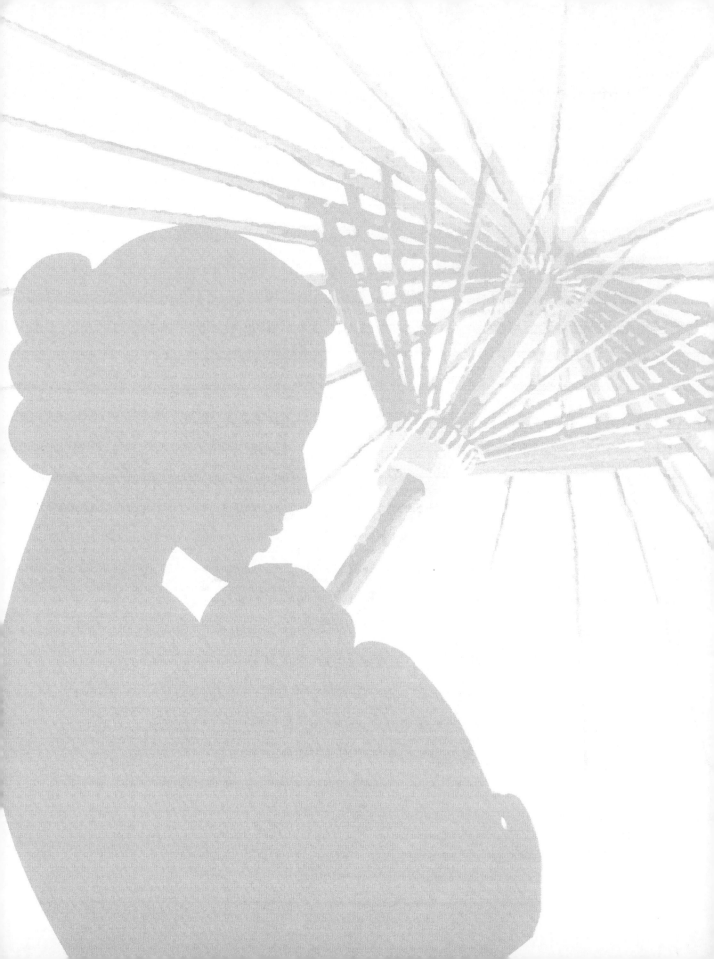

Chapter 1
Defining the Problem

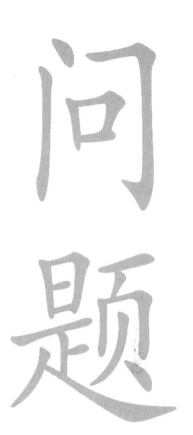

"Get pregnant. It'll fix it." conventional wisdom

The new mother lies in bed. Her belly is swaddled and she is warmly tucked in, protected from the outside world by blankets and loving family and friends who cook her meals, care for her baby, and otherwise tend to her. Her body is sore and generally out of sorts, but her heart is full of joy. She knows she will recover. Over the next month she will eat special foods and rites will be meticulously observed to protect her baby's entrance into the world.

The month after childbirth holds a sacred space in traditional cultures. They hold specific rituals and prepare special foods. Mother and child are kept protected and encouraged to rest. These are not just quaint traditions. Childbirth, and the recovery from it, is a precarious time in a woman and her newborn's lives. In premodern times high numbers of women died in childbirth and children died in infancy. Thus, every care had to be taken to maximize the health of both mother and child during this time.

Juxtapose the above experience with what many modern women experience. Overloaded with information, assistance, and medical care during their pregnancy, after delivery women disappear. Suddenly they find themselves with a new body, different from the pregnancy body but certainly not their old body either. But there is no time to worry about this. They are expected to care for the new baby 24 hours a day. Every blog, every book, every piece of advice seems focused on how the baby is developing. Is he or she latching? How long should you breast feed? Is co-sleeping better for the baby's development? What about baby sign language? Etc.

It used to be said in Western medicine that pregnancy resets a woman's hormonal balance. Perhaps this was true when women rested; and when mothers were younger. When my grandfather was practicing, a 25 year old woman having her first child was considered an "older" mom. Most of the new mothers I see in my practice are in their early 30s, and increasingly in their late 30s and in early 40s.

While pregnancy and birth are under medical supervision, modern culture has done away with postpartum care altogether. After childbirth is over there are one of two expectations: 1) women's weight, energy levels, mood, and libido, will miraculously bounce back without any assistance (just like the celebrities) or 2) women's bodies are wrecked by childbearing and any problems are "normal."

There are a whole litany of symptoms that have come to be regarded as normal after giving birth, most of which are avoidable and others which are treatable. If a woman voices her concerns about her body she is often told that it is normal and dismissed or she is judged. Traditional Chinese Medicine (TCM) would regard these as signs of imbalance. They are what I term "normal pathology." These symptoms are briefly discussed below.

Common Short and Long-term Complications of Childbirth:

Hemorrhoids

Hemorrhoids are swollen veins at or near the anus. There may be symptoms of bright red anal bleeding, a downbearing sensation, pain, and protrusion of the anus. They are a common complaint during pregnancy and after birth. The pressure of the fetus, pushing during delivery, complications of vaginal and anal tearing during delivery, constipation, and laxity in the abdomen and pelvic floor muscles after birth can all contribute to hemorrhoids. In TCM terms hemorrhoids are caused by a number of imbalances. Qi deficiency is the most common postpartum; either due to a deficiency of the upbearing function of Qi or the Qi's ability to hold Blood in the vessels. Blood stagnation is also aggravated postpartum and can cause more

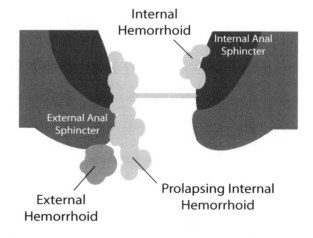

Figure 1.1. Hemorrhoids

painful and serious hemorrhoids. Damp-Heat is also a cause, but not specific to the postpartum period, unless triggered by Qi deficiency. Herbal formulas, dietary and lifestyle practices, and care during delivery help prevent them from occurring and can remedy less severe hemorrhoids. Severe hemorrhoids occasionally require surgery.

Uterine Prolapse

Uterine prolapse occurs when the network of lower abdominal and pelvic floor muscles, fascia, and ligaments that hold the uterus in place become weakened or damaged. The uterus begins to weigh down on, and eventually protrude from, the vaginal opening. The physical pressure of the uterus on other organs can cause urinary incontinence, constipation, pain during intercourse, and discomfort or a downbearing sensation in the lower abdomen. In the American population, about 40% of women develop Stage II uterine prolapse (where the uterus descends to the hymen) in their lifetime.[1] What is tragic about this statistic is that it is largely preventable with proper pelvic floor strengthening and early intervention. The most common causes are trauma to the pelvic region during childbirth, inadequate care in the month after birth, and weakened muscle tone. Uterine prolapse can occur soon after birth, but most often is a long-term complication that does not show itself until a woman is postmenopausal. In TCM, organ prolapse is a symptom of Qi deficiency; specifically a weakness of the upbearing function of Qi. Much of the focus of postpartum care is to avoid uterine prolapse.

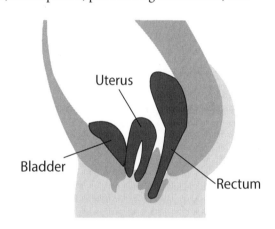

Figure 1.2. Uterine Prolapse

Pelvic Congestion Syndrome

Pelvic Congestion Syndrome refers to varicose veins in the lower abdomen. Women with this condition will feel a dull, consistent ache in the lower abdomen that worsens around menses and intercourse. This condition most commonly occurs after pregnancy. In TCM terms, Pelvic Congestion Syndrome, like varicose veins, is due to a combination of Qi deficiency (upbearing and holding functions) with Blood stasis. As the herbal medicine, diet, and lifestyle advocated in the Postpartum Recovery Program™ seek to balance Qi and Blood disorders, they will help resolve the underlying cause. They can be used successfully in conjunction with Western medical interventions.

---

1. J Eric Jelovsek. (2014). *Pelvic Organ Prolapse in Women: Choosing a Primary Surgical Procedure.* Retrieved from www. uptodate.com/contents/pelvic-organ-prolapse-in-women-choosing-a-primary-surgical-procedure

Urinary Incontinence

Urinary incontinence is the inability to control the flow of urine. There are many potential causes of urinary incontinence. Symptoms can arise immediately after birth or develop many years after. In the U.S., 33% of women over 60 suffer from incontinence.[2] After birth, it is most often due to a weakened pelvic floor. In TCM terms, urinary incontinence postpartum is most often due to a weakening of Spleen and Kidney Qi.

Diastasis Recti (Abdominal Separation)

Diastasis recti is the tearing of the linea alba; the connective tissue that joins the right and left halves of the rectus abdominis muscle. It is a common complication during the last trimester of pregnancy due to pressure from the growing fetus. Women can reduce their risks by wearing a supportive band under their abdomens during the last trimester. Wearing a postpartum girdle will speed healing of damage to the abdomen after birth. (Healing diastasis recti is discussed on page 88).

Vaginal Tearing During Childbirth

Vaginal and internal tissue tearing is a common occurrence during vaginal childbirth. This can cause long-term damage such as adhesions, nerve damage, organ prolapse, urinary or fecal incontinence, pain during intercourse, and changes in the appearance of the external genitals. Minor tears that do not involve muscles or nerves can heal quickly. Major tears can be life altering. Vaginal stretching and massage before and during birth are the traditional ways to minimize tears. There are products such as the Epi-No that uses a balloon-like device to incrementally stretch the birth canal.[3] The medical intervention is to perform an episiotomy, an incision to the vagina during birth, the benefits of which are hotly debated both amongst laywomen and physicians.

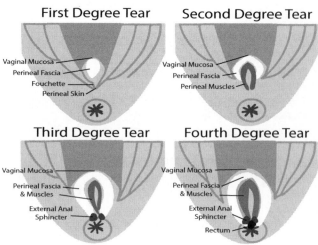

Figure 1.3. Degrees of Vaginal Tearing

2. Hannestad Y.S., Rortveit G., Sandvik H., Hunskaar S. A community-based epidemiological survey of female urinary incontinence: The Norwegian EPINCONT Study. J Clin Epidemiol 2000; 53: 1150–7.

3. Available at www.epi-no.com.au

No Libido

There are physical reasons that impede intercourse after delivery. Women should take 4-6 weeks to recover their pelvic floor and abdomen and recoup Qi and Blood before having intercourse. However, apart from the physical recovery, many women lose their sexual desire after childbirth and never regain it. There are no reliable studies on how many women suffer from lack of libido after childbirth. Anecdotally, from what patients share with me, it is rampant. There are a variety of factors: exhaustion, unresolved physical changes, depleted sex hormone levels, feeling overwhelmed with childcare and duties, and lack of emotional connection with a partner. In TCM terms postpartum low libido is most likely due to Qi and Blood deficiency. Women often become Qi and Blood deficient after giving birth and with breast feeding (which correlates with a decrease in hormones). Qi and Blood deficiency causes feelings of unattractiveness, withdrawal, and lack of desire. Without proper postpartum care, this depletion can become permanent.

Irregular Menstrual Cycle

Many women experience drastic changes to their menstruation months after they give birth. There may be amenorrhea (lack of periods), menorrhagia (excessive and irregular uterine bleeding), irregularity, and increased PMS. There are many patterns that can cause these, most of which are avoided by postpartum care, while others require more focused herbal and acupuncture treatment.

Fainting while Breast Feeding

Some women pass out when breastfeeding. This is a symptom of severe Qi and Blood deficiency. These women require herbal formulas in addition to proper postpartum care.

Stretch Marks, Sagging Abdomen and Breasts

After giving birth and breast feeding the abdomen and breasts can lose elasticity and plumpness. Though not a medical condition, this can be devastating to a woman's identity. In TCM terms this is a result of a depletion Qi and Blood (and hormone levels) as well as improper care during pregnancy and postpartum. These symptoms can be largely minimized or avoided by keeping the abdomen moisturized during pregnancy and postpartum, wearing a supportive band during the last trimester, wearing a postpartum girdle after birth, proper breast care, and following the postpartum recovery diet and lifestyle directives to recover hormonal balance (see Section II).

Weight Gain

It is a common complaint after pregnancy for women to experience stubborn weight gain. After childbirth women retain water. Unless this fluid retention is quickly dispersed it will turn to fat. Proper diet postpartum rids the body of excess fluids, resolves Dampness, strengthens Spleen Qi, and regulates the hormones helping women achieve and maintain optimal weight.

Insomnia

In addition to being woken up by their infant, many women develop long-term insomnia after giving birth. This is most often due to Qi and Blood deficiency, though it can be caused by Yin deficiency or Blood stasis as well.

Spontaneous Sweating, Night Sweats and Hot Flashes

When the Qi is weak, the body loses its ability to close the pores appropriately, leading to random sweating. This is a very common postpartum symptom. Night sweats refer to waking up hot and sweaty. Hot flashes are sudden, random waves of heat experienced throughout the day. Traditionally, it is said that pregnant women are Yang (run hot) and postpartum women are Yin (run cold). Some women, however, bypass Blood deficiency and go straight to Yin deficiency, demonstrating a more severe depletion. In Western terms, this corresponds to a more severe drop in hormones which approximates the menopausal experience.

Premature Aging

Without proper postpartum care women can experience increased wrinkles, loss of skin tone, and lingering hyperpigmentation (dark spots). This is due to Jing loss along with Qi deficiency and Blood stasis.

Low Energy/Exhaustion

Many women experience low energy due to Qi and Blood deficiency.

Disappointment and Isolation

This is a cultural symptom rather than a physical one that many women experience and it is often unspoken. For some women there is a let-down after the high expectation of birth and motherhood. Our culture does not encourage women to maintain an identity apart from being a mother. Furthermore, modern women often must choose between staying with their kids and being isolated or working to pay for daycare and feeling guilty and overworked. This was not the case for the vast majority of human history; that women must choose between social isolation and shortchanging their children. It is a social question that requires discussion. Society sets women up to complete certain milestones that we are told will fulfill us: our wedding day, motherhood, etc. These events are only fulfilling if they arise from an internal instinct and not as externally imposed expectations.

Postpartum Depression

After the above list of common symptoms, unhappiness seems like a logical addition. Women who become depleted will also be prone to depression. Women tend towards Qi and Blood deficiency with Blood stasis after childbirth. If untreated this produces low immunity, emotional sensitivity, insomnia, and depression. Excessive caretaking, which is often expected of women and mothers in particular, further depletes Qi and Blood. More severe cases of emotional instability involve Blood stasis or Phlegm obstruction.

Defining a New Normal

It is time to create a new tradition. If a woman is healthy and receives proper care and rest during the month postpartum she can expect to be renewed after childbirth. Her hormones and natural rhythms are reset. Her waistline returns to normal gradually over a three month period and her figure will return to pre-pregnancy or better. Lochia stops after two weeks (four at most). Menstruation returns after four months. Her hair and skin retain their tone and luster. Her breasts and vaginal area recover after six months to a year.

The horrible trick that is played on women is that they go into pregnancy expecting this outcome without the tools to make it a reality. Instead they think there is something horribly wrong with them when it does not. Or else they believe that pregnancy and childbirth are supposed to be damaging and to complain will only bring judgment upon them. The cure for shame is speaking out, and the cure for ignorance is education. In the next chapters we will discuss the theory behind postpartum care and then present the full Postpartum Recovery Program™. This book will teach you how to rejuvenate your hormones, how to maintain your strength as a woman, and stay happy. Your baby will be at his/her best when you are.

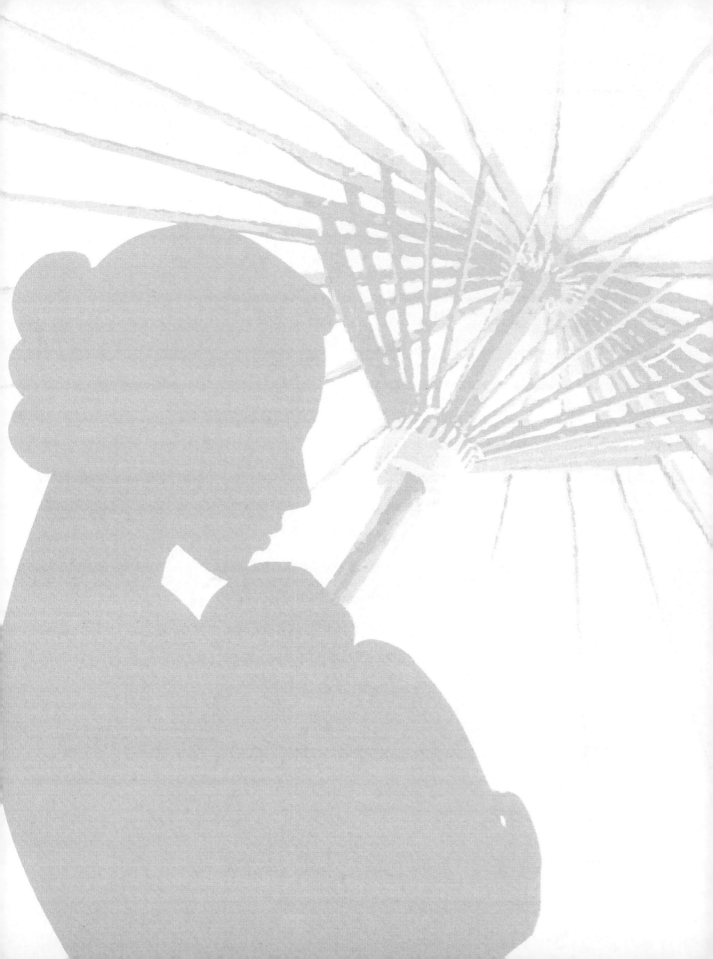

Chapter 2
Traditional Chinese Medicine

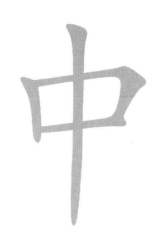

It is Chiang Mai, Thailand, as the end of the world nears in December 2012. I sit comfortably in a large octagon-shaped room with a Thai banana in my hand and cozy slippers warming my toes from the blasting air conditioning. The room is encircled with porcelain figurines of Daoist sages collected by Master Mantak Chia. It is a class on Chinese astrology and I listen as Master Chia meanders from one topic to the next, as masters often do, following a logical progression apparent only to them. Finally, after finishing a personal lament on Metal Tiger women making difficult wives, he insightfully ties all of Traditional Chinese Medicine (TCM)[1] and Daoism[2] into a simple concept.

I will paraphrase. Daoism explains humanity's complicated situation thusly: we stand between Heaven and Earth. We are made of both, connected to both, and constantly harmonize these two opposites. We are given both predetermined circumstances and things we can change. Traditionally, a person would have his or her astrological chart read. This determines one's "Heaven luck;" the strengths and weaknesses we have been endowed with by birth. These are unchangeable, but we

---

1. TCM in this book refers to the traditional medicine of China and its modern practice throughout the world. It was born at least 2,500 years ago, alongside the religious philosophies of Daoism, Confucianism, and Buddhism.

2. Daoism is a native religious philosophy of China created over 2,500 years ago. Daoism gave TCM the concepts of Yin and Yang, the 5 Elements, and other foundational principles so that it is difficult to separate the two.

can learn to make the most of them. Qigong, nutrition, and other aspects of self-cultivation are considered our "Human luck." This is the good fortune we create by our determination and our choices. Then we have Feng Shui which is our "Earth luck." It allows us to modify our environment to maximize what we need and neutralize what is not helpful.

The practice of TCM concerns itself with "Human luck." It seeks to map out natural cycles in relation to our personal strengths and weaknesses. This allows us to carry out practical strategies that will increase our heath, youthfulness, and virtue.

Learning a New Language

Western science chose to approach the issue of paradox by doing away with extraneous information and reducing the world into limited pieces of absolute truth. A scientific study is designed to minimize variables in order to analyze the effects of a single factor, such as whether or not a specific medication at a specific dose alleviates migraine headaches. A western practitioner then mimics the treatment strategy that proves effective in most cases of migraine headaches. Asian science chose to keep the whole picture intact and to accept the inevitable complications. The focus in Asian science has been on how individual pieces relate within the whole. For example, in order to assess the efficacy of medicinals for a migraine headache, numerous factors need to be taken into consideration. A TCM practitioner might ask: What is the constitution of the patient? What is their health history, diet, and lifestyle? Is headache frequency and severity influenced by seasonal or hormonal cycles? The end result is a more complicated amassment of data, which leads to a treatment strategy more specific to the individual patient.

To the ancient Chinese, a scholar was a Renaissance man; versed in art, science, physical culture, and philosophy. An educated Chinese person was judged until recently not only on the number of Chinese characters he or she knew, but also on the ability to write them beautifully. Thus, Chinese medicine developed as an integration of right and left brain observations. The language of the traditional medicine of China contains multiple levels of meaning, as the physician was expected to treat multiple levels of health – physical, emotional, mental, and spiritual.

It is easy to get lost in the poetry of TCM language when you first hear it. I remember being enthralled when my professor in an introductory class used phrases like the "violent marauding of blood" and "the Liver attacks the Stomach causing Qi rebellion." You might be tempted to dismiss its validity, coming from a world that values technical language. However, the benefit of metaphorical language is that it allows for layered meaning and the existence of paradox. The deeper we delve into the physical, emotional, mental, and spiritual health of humans, the more we will be confronted with contradiction.

For example, if I use technical language to tell you that you need to strengthen your pelvic floor muscles, it leads to anatomical diagrams and Kegel exercises. However, if I tell you that you need to conserve your Jing and that one of the leakage points for Jing is a point at your perineum, it opens up a discussion on physical muscle development in a much greater context. TCM gives us the ability to focus mental energy, to understand how we are talking about more than keeping your urine and uterus from leaking out. It is about revitalizing your entire endocrine system and physical power. Additionally, it relates how this strength translates into balancing your emotions and mind, all of which facilitate spiritual practice.

TCM 's view on postpartum care is as relevant today as it has ever been. The Postpartum Recovery Program™ does not fight modern care of pregnancy and birth. It enhances it. To say there is only one science to describe the totality of the natural world is like saying there is one language that voices everything we as humans want to express. Different languages excel in certain areas and fall short in others. TCM is able to explain the subtleties of postpartum changes in a way Western medicine cannot.

Following Nature, Intelligently

Thousands of years of Daoist inquiry concluded that being in sync with nature heals us, and living contrary to nature causes disease. To follow natural cycles you should wake up early with the sun. Have your strongest activity, eat your biggest meals, and do your most intense mental work between 6:00 a.m. and early afternoon. Eat less, relax, and connect in late afternoon and evening. Go to bed at 10:00 p.m. and sleep until 6:00 or 7:00 a.m. Detox and begin new ventures in the spring. Sleep late, have too much fun, and expand in the summer. Take an inventory of your goals and strategize your next move during the fall. Rest more and turn inward in the winter. Whenever we feel lost, overworked or scattered, we need only sit in nature. It will bring us back in harmony with natural cycles. If you spend a lot of time in traffic or around electronic devices, balance it with exposure to the natural world. Listen to the birds, take a walk in the woods, tend your garden, daydream by a lake, or play with your pets.

To think one can compete with or overtake nature is foolish. It is to compete against ourselves. We are part of nature. Just as surely as we are animated by spirit and connected to the heavens, we are animals made of water sustained by food grown on the earth. We are just as influenced by the moon as is the tide. Understanding this is the secret to vitality.

This is not to say that we should do whatever we want, whenever we want, and all will be well. The philosophies that influenced TCM, Daoism, Confucianism, and Buddhism, all agree that humans are the composite of various elements. We are naturally virtuous, good, and act in a health-affirming manner when we balance and cultivate ourselves. We are naturally destructive when we are unbalanced. Thus qigong, meditation, lifestyle, and nutritional practices were developed in order to keep us balanced so that we could rely on our inner guidance to make the right choices for the betterment of ourselves and society.

The Trouble with Babies and Baby-Making

There are a few areas of life that tend to get us into trouble. Perhaps most notably is procreation and the drive behind it. Socially, sexuality without the bounds of morality creates chaos. But more important to ancient Daoists was the observation that unconscious sexual expression and procreation was a waste of our genetic material (or Jing, described below). Men lose genetic material through ejaculation; thus men can increase their vitality by limiting ejaculation and becoming conscious in their sexuality.[3] Women lose genetic material during menstruation and childbearing; thus women increase vitality by following special practices during menses and during the month after giving birth. Genetic material naturally begins to wane by the time women are about 35, and men about 40, depending on their genetics and how they live their lives. Men and women should begin rejuvenation practices at 35 and 40, respectively, in preparation for menopause and andropause.[4] With age, women tend towards Yin deficiency, men towards Yang deficiency.

Besides depleting Jing, childbirth and breastfeeding create the tendency towards Qi and Blood deficiency with Blood stasis (these terms are described below). Qi is injured during delivery and is further taxed by the demands of healing postpartum. Childbirth brings significant blood and fluid loss. Additionally, breast milk production is considered analogous to blood production. Postpartum women must thoroughly pass the residual blood and tissue from the uterus in the weeks after birth, known as lochia. It is easy for this process to be interrupted and for residual tissue to remain in the uterus causing potential uterine dysfunction in the future.

Historically, when the value of women was not held very high, it was still considered critical to optimize women's health for the sake of the lineage. The ancient Chinese understood, by means of recorded observation, that the genetic material of both parents dictates what future generations will inherit. Modern epigenetics research shows that not just DNA, but alterations to the genome due to personal experiences can alter the genetics of generations to come. For example, famine experienced by a grandparent can lead to increased propensity towards diabetes or shorter lifespan in a grandchild.[5]

Sacredness of Womanhood

The Huichol[6] believe women, by virtue of the physicality of their cycles are more connected with nature, and it is the job of women to keep men, who do not have such reminders, in harmony with their surroundings.[7] TCM similarly values women's cycles. In addition to being a physical reminder of our link with nature, menstrual, postpartum, and menopausal symptoms are precise indicators of imbalance in the body. Honor your cycles as a great blessing and listen to your symptoms.

---

3. Men are socialized subtly, and not so subtly, to separate sexuality from emotions and spirituality. They are encouraged to harden their hearts, follow base instincts, to "spread their seed", "sow their wild oats", and to rely on pornography, all of which focus vital energy outwards.

4. Andropause refers to a decline in sex hormones in men that occurs around middle age and is associated with a decline in muscles tone, sexual virility, fertility, and an increase in irritability and depression.

5. Based on what is known as the Överkalix study. For more see: Whitelaw, Emma. Sins of the fathers, and their fathers. European Journal of Human Genetics (2006) 14, 131–132. doi:10.1038/sj.ejhg.5201567

6. Or Wixáritari, are a Native American tribe originating in the Sierra Madre Occidental range in Mexico.

7. An anonymous Huichol source.

The Three Treasures: Qi, Shen, & Jing

If Jing and Qi are healthy and flourishing, the Shen will be happy and this will lead to a healthy and happy life.

TCM Principle

The three treasures are vital substances in the body which TCM considers the most important to keep balanced.

气 Qì; Our Strength

The traditional character for Qi is 氣. It contains the radical 米 (mǐ) which means "rice," contained within the radical 气 which depicts steam rising from the rice. Rice holds a near sacred symbolism in Chinese culture. It was the staple grain in the majority of the country, thus having rice meant sustenance. Qi is the rarified energy released from this perfect food when cooked. This gives us a clear visual about the nature of Qi. It has a warm, upward rising, insubstantial nature.

Qi is sometimes translated as "life force" or "vital energy." It fuels all of the functions of the body. Qi is damaged during delivery and much of the focus of the Postpartum Recovery Program™ is rehabilitating the Qi.

> **THE STATE OF OUR QI TELLS US:**
> 1. Our ability to digest food and life experiences.
> 2. Our energy levels.
> 3. The strength and development of our muscles.

Functions of Qi:
Transforming, transporting, holding, raising, protecting, and warming.

Signs of Qi Deficiency:
Pale complexion, organ prolapse, edema, spider veins, loose stools, abdominal bloating and fatigue (especially after meals), poor absorption, spontaneous sweating, weak digestion, timidity, foggy head, muscle weakness, flabby skin, poor muscle tone, short menstrual cycle, heavy bleeding, pale menstrual blood.

Things that Deplete Qi:
Physical overwork, excessive weightlifting, fasting, extreme dieting, extreme sweating, excessive cold or raw foods.

Things that Tonify Qi:
Regular rest, warming easily digestible diet.

Signs of Qi Stagnation:

Irritability, mood swings, abdominal bloating, PMS, irregular menstrual cycle, breast distention, insufficient lactation (blocked), constipation or alternating constipation and diarrhea, IBS.

Things that Stagnate Qi:

Emotional stress, environmental toxins, medications, poor diet, irregular sleep, Qi deficiency.

Things that Move Qi:

Exercise, qigong, tai chi, yoga, pungent flavors or smells, regular sleep and diet.

神 Shén; Our Consciousness

The character for Shen is the combination of 礻 (示 shì) meaning "altar" and 申 shēn which gives the phonetic pronunciation. Shen can be used to mean "spirit" in a variety of contexts. Each of the twelve main organ systems has its own spirit or Shen. The Shen is also used to describe the overall spirit of the body. Shen is best described as "consciousness." The Shen is housed in the Blood. When the Blood becomes deficient, as is the tendency postpartum, the Shen loses its home and becomes disturbed.

> **THE STATE OF OUR SHEN TELLS US:**
> 1. If we behave appropriately.
> 2. How we handle intimacy.
> 3. Our level of consciousness.

Functions of Shen:
Awareness of self, integration of emotions, connection with others, love.

Signs of Shen Disturbance:
Postpartum depression, lack of bonding with the newborn, insomnia, irrational thinking and behavior, inappropriate laughing or crying.

Things that Disturb the Shen:
Emotional trauma, abuse, abandonment, heartbreak, physical or emotional exhaustion, Blood or Yin deficiency, Phlegm, Blood stasis.

Things that Calm the Shen:
Relaxing music, peaceful environment, being nurtured.

精 Jīng; Our Genetic Inheritance

The character for Jing contains the "rice" radical 米 (mǐ) and 青 (qīng) which gives the phonetic pronunciation. 青 (qīng) also connotes the color of nature, youthfulness, and things not yet ripe; thus a vital potential as yet unleashed. Jing is a difficult concept to grasp in the West, but understanding it is essential to understanding why Postpartum Recovery is so critical. In a way, Jing is opposite to the Qi and Shen. Where they are insubstantial, Jing is pure substance. It is the genetic and hormonal matter concentrated in our bone marrow, cerebral spinal fluid, endocrine organs, and brain that forms the foundation of our physical vitality.

Jing can be divided into Pre-Heaven Jing (our inherited potential), Post-Heaven Jing (vitality based on life choices), and Jing (the combination of Pre and Post-Heaven).

Pre-Heaven Jing (Genetic Destiny)

Pre-Heaven Jing is our inherited potential. It is created at conception, when the sexual energies from both parents unite. In utero, the Po, the Yin aspect of the soul, uses the Jing to create the matrix of the body. [8] This matrix contains the information for our unique physical expression and divines how we will develop, if we will reproduce, when we will age, and when we are likely to die. After we are born, Jing moves in very slow cycles; 7 years for women and 8 years for men. Somewhere in our late thirties and early forties Jing weakens and the matrix becomes increasingly disordered, leading us to eventual death.

We cannot generate Pre-Heaven Jing. All we can do is keep the genetic material from leaking out. Pre-Heaven Jing is conserved when we live a balanced life, and depleted when we live excessively (too much work, play, drugs, sex, children, stress, and excitement without enough rest). We have no control over what we inherit. Pre-Heaven Jing is like destiny. We do not choose our destiny but we can choose to live in accordance with it or against it.

Post-Heaven Jing (Free Will)

Post-Heaven Jing is generated from our diet and the air we breathe, and thus controlled to a large extent by our daily choices. It is associated with the health of the Spleen and Stomach systems (digestion) and the Lungs. Much of the focus of the Postpartum Recovery Program™, and TCM as a whole, is on maximizing Post-Heaven Jing. Living a balanced life in accordance with daily and seasonal cycles, eating well, practicing breathing techniques, and managing stress all increase Post-Heaven Jing. Energy cultivation practices such as qigong and tai chi focus on protecting and generating Jing.[9] This is the piece where we have control over our destiny.

Unfortunately our ability to generate Post-Heaven Jing becomes limited in a polluted environment and with degraded quality of food and air. Naturally grown foods have the most Qi. Without

---

8. Giovanni Maciocia. *The Psyche in Chinese Medicine; Treatment of Emotional and Mental Disharmonies with Acupuncture and Chinese Herbs.* (Nanjing: Churchill Livingstone, 2009), 48.

9. Qigong (气功, Wade–Giles: chi kung) literally means "Qi exercise." It includes a wide variety of practices dating back over 4,000 years in China that were used in martial arts schools, Daoist cultivation, Buddhist practice, and Confucianism. The general purpose of qigong is to strengthen and calm the mind, increase health and longevity, and improve mind-body connection. Examples of qigong include: meditation, dao-in (yoga-like exercises), 6 healing sounds (similar to mantra), 5 animal frolics (animal-inspired movements), and standing meditation. Tai chi (太極拳, *tài jí quán*) can be considered a form of qigong, using breath and a complex, graceful choreography. It developed as an internal martial art, but now is mostly used for health and stress relief.

artificial help or machines, plants and animals will only produce well when farmers follow natural rhythms, rotate crops, and offer livestock a healthy environment. It is not only the improved quality of naturally grown foods, it is also how the act of producing quality foods improves us. Natural farming forces farmers to be in tune with natural cycles and to become acutely aware when patterns are off.[10]

Factory farming methods, genetically modified seeds, and massive dependence on pesticides create a false sense of separation from our environment and produce foods that cause digestive and endocrine disturbances[11] and provide us with less Qi. Factory farming raises animals in stressful and inhumane conditions, the energy and diseases of which get passed along in dairy and meat products. Thus they do not nourish us the same way naturally grown food do. Food is the first medicine and it is vitally important for us to protect our food supply. When we honor the land and cultivate food with respect we produce superior food. The environment and humanity both benefit.

The second major way we receive energy and Post-Heaven Jing from our environment is through breathing. Qigong, meditation, yoga, and tai chi practices all utilize the power of the breath to rejuvenate and center us. These benefits are diminished as we breathe increasingly toxic air.

Besides disrupting our ability to build Jing, it appears that environmental toxicity is increasingly affecting our Jing directly. We can see evidence of this in hormonal disruption and diminished sperm and egg quality directly caused by pollutants. Women appear to be experiencing more fertility issues, as evidenced by the growing number of physicians and acupuncturists catering to infertility. This is due not only to women having babies older, but also to toxic exposure and chronic stress.[12] For example, there are numerous studies on the negative effects of bisphenol-A (BPA), commonly used in plastic bottles and in the lining of canned foods, on fertility and metabolic functioning of males and females.[13] A 1992 British study showed that male sperm quality has declined since the mid-1900s.[14] Rising rates of infertility and a decrease in the quality of eggs and sperm are a clear sign of increasing Jing insufficiency in humans. This impacts the quality of our health and that of future generations. Thus reducing emotional stress and environmental pollution on a personal and global level needs to be a priority for us all.

---

10. For example, I have heard many historical references to longevity and vitality being attributed to having hives and consuming bee products such as honey, propolis, and royal jelly. Having worked with bees I believe it is the act of lovingly maintaining a hive that creates longevity, more than consuming the hive products. The energy of the bees is incredible and simply being in their space is energizing. Bees are also highly responsive to vibration. If you are disrespectful, stressed out, afraid, or in a rush when working with them they will give you immediate, and dramatic, feedback. Thus they offer an excellent reminder to keep your mind calm.

11. For example a recent study suggests that the rise in gluten sensitivities may be due in part to exposure to glyphosate, the main ingredient in Roundup, a prevalent pesticide. Samsel, Anthony, and Seneff, Stephanie. (2013), Glyphosate, Pathways to Modern Diseases II: Celiac Sprue and Gluten Intolerance. Interdiscip Toxicol. 2013; Vol. 6 (4): 159–184. doi: 10.2478/intox-2013-0026

12. Petraglia F1, Serour GI, Chapron C. (2013), The Changing Prevalence of Infertility. Int J Gynaecol Obstet - December 2013 (Vol. 123, Suppl 2:S4-8). doi: 10.1016/j.ijgo.2013.09.005. Epub 2013 Sep 7.

13. Fenichel P1, Chevalier N, Brucker-Davis F. (2013), Bisphenol A: An Endocrine and Metabolic Disruptor. Ann Endocrinol (Paris) - July 2013 (Vol. 74, Issue3, Pages 211-20). doi: 10.1016/j.ando.2013.04.002. Epub 2013 Jun 21.

14. E. Carlsen, A. Giwercman, N. Keiding and N.E. Skakkebaek. (1992), Evidence for Decreasing Quality of Semen During the Past 50 Years. British Medical Journal -1992 (Vol. 305, N° 6854, Pages 609-613).

Jing

The term "Jing" includes both inherited Jing (Pre-Heaven) and the effects of our lifestyle choices (Post-Heaven). Jing is stored in the Kidneys and sexual organs and circulates throughout the body. Jing is lost through reproduction; through ejaculation in men, and menstruation and childbirth in women. This is why conscious ejaculation practices in men and menstrual and postpartum care in women are critical for maximizing our genetics and changing how we age.

Women not only lose blood every month, we also lose our genetic material in the form of an egg or two. If we become pregnant, the growing fetus draws upon our Kidney energy (Jing) during gestation.[15] Delivery and breastfeeding further tax the body. Women should space childbirth by 2-3 years to allow time for full recovery in between.[16] The quality of recovery is just as important as the time. Women should practice the Postpartum Recovery Program™ during the first 30-40 days after birth. There is an additional issue; the value of quality over quantity in terms of child-bearing. Less children means each child receives more resources from his/her parents. The mother has more Jing available to offer each fetus, and parents can invest more time and resources towards each child. Chinese and Taiwanese cultures place a high value on family and preparing each child to excel in life.

> ### THE STATE OF OUR JING TELLS US:
>
> 1. When and how we will age.
>
> 2. If we can reproduce.
>
> 3. Whether or not we can ward off disease or survive hardship.

The concept of Jing brings up the issue of older parents. The modern trend is for people to wait to have children. This is beneficial in that more mature and financially stable parents have more to offer their children. However, older parents have less Jing, or genetic material, to pass on to their offspring.[17] This issue is widely accepted for older mothers who have increased risks of bearing children with Down syndrome and other genetic abnormalities.[18] There are a number of studies that also link older fathers to increased genetic abnormalities in children such as schizophrenia[19] and

---

15. Some mothers would argue it does not stop at gestation, but rather mothers continue to give of themselves to their children for the rest of their lives as suggested in a 2006 Polish study: Grazyna Jasienska, Ilona Nenko, and Michal Jasienski. (2006), Daughters Increase Longevity of Fathers, but Daughters and Sons Equally Reduce Longevity of Mothers. American Journal Of Human Biology - 2006 (Vol. 18, Pages 422–425).

16. There have been numerous studies linking bearing and rearing offspring to shortened lifespans in females. When the intervals between offspring is shortened, life expectancy reduces more dramatically: Mühlbock, O. (1959), Factors Influencing the Lifespan of Inbred Mice. Gerontologica – 1959 (Vol. 3, Pages 177-183) and Murray, W.S. (1965), Biological Significance of Factors Influencing the Incidence of Mammary Cancer in Mice. J. Nat. Cancer Inst. – 1965 (Vol. 34, Pages 21-41).

17. Menopause is brought on by Jing deficiency. As women near menopause they have declining levels of Jing to pass on to children. Of course this varies widely based on genetics and self-care practices. Men undergo a similar process beginning at age 40 and declining Jing levels eventually trigger andropause.

18. Mary Esther Gaulden. (1992), Maternal Age Effect: The Enigma of Down Syndrome and Other Trisomic Conditions. Mutation Research/Reviews in Genetic Toxicology - December 1992 (Volume 296, Issues 1–2, Pages 69–88). doi: 10.1016/0165-1110(92)90033-6

19. Malaspina, D., Corcoran, C., Fahim, C., Berman, A., Harkavy-Friedman, J., Yale, S., Goetz, D., Goetz, R., Harlap, S. and Gorman, J. (2002), Paternal age and sporadic schizophrenia: Evidence for de novo mutations. Am. J. Med. Genet., 114: 299–303. doi: 10.1002/ajmg.1701

autism.[20] Interestingly, the age at which genetic abnormalities increase is in fathers 40 and over,[21] the exact age the Yellow Emperor's Inner Canon claims men's Jing begins to decline.[22] Although men produce new sperm throughout their lifetime, the quality of their sperm is dependent on the current state of their Jing.

Having less Jing also means that women will have a more difficult time recovering from childbirth. The Postpartum Recovery Program™ becomes even more critical in women 35 years or older to preserve Jing and improve the health of their infants (through quality breast milk).

Signs of Jing deficiency:
Poor development or mental impairment in children, infertility, habitual miscarriage, bone loss, loose teeth, hair loss, premature graying, poor sexual function, weak knees, tinnitus, deafness, poor concentration, poor memory, dizziness, frequent colds, and chronic rhinitis.

Factors that Deplete Jing:
Physical and mental overwork, chronic emotional stress, drug and alcohol abuse, bearing several children or children spaced too closely together, and excessive sex.

Factors that Conserve Jing:
Balance between rest and activity, living in harmony with natural cycles, tai chi, and qigong. In women, proper menstrual, postpartum, and menopausal care. In men, conscious ejaculation methods.

20. Reichenberg A, Gross R, Weiser M, et al. Advancing Paternal Age and Autism. Arch Gen Psychiatry. 2006;63(9):1026-1032. doi:10.1001/archpsyc.63.9.1026

21. Friedman, J M. (1981), Genetic Disease in the Offspring of Older Fathers. Obstetrics & Gynecology - June 1981 (Vol. 57, Issue 6, Pages 745-749).

22. The Yellow Emperor's Inner Canon (黄帝内经 *Huángdì Nèijīng*) is thought to have been written between the late Warring States period (475-221 BC) and the early Han period (206 BCE–220 CE) in China. It is the first written record of acupuncture and TCM theory. It is considered a foundational text in TCM and Daoist philosophy. The first chapter describes the 7 year cycles of Jing for women and 8 year cycles of Jing for men. The topic of women's Jing cycles is covered in Andrews, Lia. *7 Times a Woman; Ancient Wisdom on Health & Beauty for Every Stage of Your Life*. (Alcyone Press: San Diego, 2013).

Other Vital Substances

血 Blood (*xuè*); Our Substance

The term "blood" in TCM encompasses more than the Western concept. Blood is the physical manifestation of Qi and is inseparable from it. Qi gives life to the Blood, while Blood gives Qi physical form. Blood is nourishing and moistening. The health of the Spleen, and to a lesser extent Kidneys, Lungs, and Heart, are crucial for Blood production. Blood is ruled by the Heart and stored in the Liver. Blood loss is a characteristic of childbirth and the ensuing lochial discharge. Blood is also associated with breast milk and healthy milk production requires strong Blood. For these reasons all postpartum women tend towards Blood deficiency and should nourish Blood as a preventive measure.

Signs of Blood Deficiency:
Pallor (pale face, pale tongue, etc.), look like the light is out, lack of glow, dry skin, dry hair, fatigue, weak nails, unstable blood sugar, scanty breast milk, watery breast milk, scanty, pale menstruation, delayed menstruation or long cycles, constipation, emotional sensitivity, poor self-image, low libido, palpitations, anxiety, timidity, depression, insomnia, foggy head.

> **THE STATE OF OUR BLOOD TELLS US:**
>
> 1. The glow and luster of our skin and hair.
>
> 2. The flexibilty of tendons and muscles, particularly of the neck and upper back.
>
> 3. Our ability to be steady and calm, rather than feeling overwhelmed and vulnerable.

Things that Deplete Blood:
Mental overwork (particularly on the computer), excessive bleeding, not resting during menses, caretaking and nourishing others.

Things that Nourish Blood:
Practicing proper menstrual care , regular rest, Blood nourishing diet, acupuncture.

Signs of Blood Stagnation:
Depression, insomnia, history of physical or emotional trauma, stuck thought patterns, menstrual cramps, dark menstrual bleeding with clots, purplish or bluish tinge to skin, visible purple veins.

Things that Stagnate Blood:
Physical trauma, accidents, unresolved emotional trauma, chronic Blood deficiency.

Things that Move Blood:
Exercise, qigong, massage, acupuncture, tai chi, yoga, pungent flavors or smells, regular sleep and diet, moxibustion.

津液 Body Fluids (*jīn yè*)

Body fluids are derived from food and drink. The Spleen separates the pure fluids and sends them to the Lungs and Kidneys, sending the impure fluids to the Small Intestines. Body fluid deficiency is grouped with Blood or Yin deficiency. Delivery and breastfeeding are taxing on body fluids and thus conserving and replenishing body fluids is an important aspect of the Postpartum Recovery Program™.

阴 Yīn; Our Feminine Principle

Yin is a much used term in Eastern thought as the counterpart to Yang to explain the duality of creation. Yin is interior, heavy, dark, and still while Yang is exterior, light, bright, and active. Harmony and health requires the balance of these two forces. In regards to the physical body, Yin represents the substance and fluids. Insufficient Yin means we are unable to quiet ourselves or look inward. It means our body lacks substance, i.e. is too thin. It means it does not have enough moisture or coolness. Clinically speaking, Yin deficiency is a progression of Blood deficiency. Compared to Blood deficiency, Yin deficiency is characterized by more fluid deficiency, more pronounced weakness, and the emergence of Heat signs.

Women, being more Yin in nature, also consume more Yin, and tend towards Yin deficiency as we age, particularly after age 35 and through perimenopause. Many modern women become Yin deficient after giving birth (without proper postpartum care). This is partly because women are having children later and because our modern lifestyle is more depleting to Yin.

> **THE STATE OF OUR YIN TELLS US:**
>
> 1. Whether or not we can settle down and stay present.
>
> 2. If we are able to be receptive and listen.
>
> 3. Our ability to stay cool; physically and figuratively.

Signs of Yin Deficiency:
Dryness (skin, eyes, vagina, hair), palpitations, scanty breast milk, thinning skin, wrinkles, heat on palms and soles of the feet, heat at night, hot flashes, night sweats, constipation, low back and knee soreness and weakness, restlessness, anxiety, insomnia, emotional instability, tinnitus, excess libido, headaches, malar flush (red cheeks), menstruation bright red, spotting, short cycles, poor memory.

Things that Deplete Yin:
Mental overwork (particularly on the computer), overstimulation, electronics and noise, many legal and illegal drugs, excess alcohol, excessive sweating (saunas, cardio, hot room yoga), smoking.

Things that Nourish Yin:
Regular rest, leisure, relaxation, cooling and moistening diet.

阳 Yáng; Our Masculine Principle

Whereas Yin represents the substance and fluids, Yang represents the action and heat of the body. Insufficient Yang means the body lacks energy to move muscles, digest food, or perform cellular reactions. It means it lacks heat to warm and mobilize the body. It means we are unable to wake up early, maintain clear focus, and have passion for life. Clinically speaking, Yang deficiency is a progression of Qi deficiency. Compared to Qi deficiency, Yang deficiency is characterized by lesser functioning, more pronounced weakness, and the emergence of Cold signs. Men tend towards Yang deficiency as they age, particularly after age 40. Some women also tend towards Yang deficiency, which can be aggravated postpartum.

> **THE STATE OF OUR YANG TELLS US:**
>
> 1. Whether or not we have the will and stamina to persevere.
> 2. If we are able to take action.
> 3. Our ability to warm up; physically and figuratively.

Signs of Yang Deficiency:
Cold feeling, pale complexion, pale urine, loose stools with undigested food, cock's crow diarrhea (loose stools first thing in the morning), edema, abdominal bloating, weak digestion, tinnitus, low back and knee soreness and weakness, low libido, late periods, prolonged bleeding and trickling after period starts.

Things that Deplete Yang:
Physical overwork, excessive weightlifting, excessive exposure to cold (deep sea diving, swimming in cold water), and excessive cold or raw foods.

Things that Tonify Yang:
Regular rest, warming diet.

Pathological Substances

风 External Wind (*fēng*)

External wind is the TCM term to describe pathogenic invasions of viral and bacterial origin such as the common cold, flu, strep throat, and sinus infection. Wind enters the body through the nose, mouth, and open pores and produces a sudden onset of symptoms. The TCM understanding of pathogenic invasion is complex and takes into consideration the strength of the body and the strength of the pathogen. Certain internal environments such as Qi and Blood deficiency (i.e. low immunity) leaves people prone to Wind Invasion. This is why Wind, and particularly Wind Cold, is such a concern for postpartum women. The Qi and Blood are depleted, immunity is low, meaning that any pathogen can move in and take hold in the body with greater ease. Wind carries in other pathogenic substances such as Cold, Heat, and Dampness.

Signs of Wind Cold:
Runny nose with clear or white mucous, cough, easily chilled, dislikes drafts, muscle aches, sinus headache, stiff neck and shoulders.

> **KEY SIGN OF EXTERNAL WIND:**
>
> Aversion to drafts and wind.

Signs of Wind Heat:
Stuffy nose with yellow mucous, cough, fever, thirst, easily chilled, sore throat, irritability, muscle aches, sinus headache, stiff neck and shoulders.

Signs of Wind Dampness:
Joint stiffness and pain, joint swelling.

Things that Cause Wind Invasion:
Exposure to cold or drafts when you are depleted, weak, or have wet clothes or hair. Not adequately covering up in cold or wet weather. Sitting on cold or damp surfaces.

Things that Treat Wind Invasion:
Sweating, pungent teas and soups, rest, acupuncture, running cupping, gua sha, Wind-dispersing herbs.

寒 Cold (*hán*)

Cold runs counter to the warm, energetic processes of the body. Cold freezes and stagnates metabolic functioning. Cold is injurious particularly to the Kidneys. It can result from deficiency of

Qi and/or Yang in the body or exposure to excessive cold can overwhelm even the strongest body. Qi deficiency that occurs due to delivery and postpartum healing predisposes women to Cold.

Signs of Cold:
Pain ameliorated by heat, aversion to cold, feeling cold, craving warm drinks or food.

Things that Cause Cold:
Exposure to cold wet weather, repeated exposure to cold water, Qi and Yang deficiency.

> **KEY SIGNS OF COLD:**
> 1. Craving warm foods and drinks.
> 2. Symptoms alleviated by warmth.

Things that Treat Cold:
Warm cooked foods, spices, high protein diet, acupuncture, moxibustion, warming herbs.

热 Heat (*rè*)

Pathological Heat translates best as "inflammation" in Western terms. This is metabolic functioning unchecked by the body's internal cooling system. It can result from deficiency of Yin in the body or exposure to excessive heat can overwhelm even the strongest body. As more women are becoming Yin deficient postpartum, Heat symptoms are becoming more prevalent.

Signs of Heat:
Pain ameliorated by cold, aversion to heat, feeling hot, redness, irritability, craving cold drinks or food, constipation, rashes or acne, inflammation, body odor, excessive sweating, high blood pressure.

> **KEY SIGNS OF HEAT:**
> 1. Craving cold foods and drinks.
> 2. Symptoms alleviated by cold.

Things that Cause Heat:
Excessive spicy foods or meat, excess alcohol, toxic exposure, Yin deficiency.

Things that Treat Heat:
Raw and cooling foods, high vegetable diet, acupuncture, cupping, gua sha, cooling herbs.

痰 Phlegm (*tán*)

The terms Phlegm and Dampness refer to congestion and accumulation of body fluids in different manifestations. The term Phlegm-Damp is used to refer to systemic or non-specific congestion and accumulation of fluids, while Phlegm and Damp might be used to indicate specific locations or symptoms. Phlegm is used to refer to the Upper Jiao (Lungs and Heart), mental impairment (as in misting the Mind, foggy thinking, irrational behavior) and in certain channel pathology.

Signs of Phlegm:
Heaviness, lethargy, runny nose, sinus congestion, productive cough, puffiness around the eyes or face, excess fat that feels hard, cellulite, foggy head, cognitive impairment, irrational thoughts or behavior, obsessive thoughts, ruminating, high cholesterol, tumors and masses, poor motor function.

> **KEY SIGNS OF PHLEGM:**
> 1. Excessive mucous production.
> 2. Lethargy.

Things that Cause Phlegm:
The root of Phlegm is poor digestion: improper diet, excessive intake of fatty or greasy foods, excess sugar intake, excess raw foods, weak digestion (Qi deficiency).

Things that Treat Phlegm:
Exercise, movement, high vegetable diet (cooked), bitter, spicy, or pungent taste or smell, acupuncture, running cupping, gua sha, lymphatic drainage (endermologie™), Phlegm-resolving herbs.

湿气 Dampness (*shī qì*)

Dampness refers to congestion and accumulation of fluids in the Middle and Lower Jiaos (mucus and bloating in the digestive tract, cloudy and dribbling urination). Dampness is injurious particularly to the Spleen (and digestion). Because Qi is weak postpartum, it is easy to develop Dampness and stubborn weight gain.

Signs of Dampness:
Heaviness, lethargy, abdominal bloating, loose stools, mucous in the stools, excess fat that feels soft or flabbiness, cellulite, edema (fluid retention), cloudy urination, white leucorrhea (vaginal discharge), worrying, not letting things go, Candida (yeast infection, thrush), joint stiffness and pain, joint swelling.

> **KEY SIGNS OF DAMPNESS:**
> 1. Water retention.
> 2. Vaginal discharge.

Things that Cause Dampness:
The root of Dampness is poor digestion: improper diet, excessive intake of fatty or greasy foods, excess sugar intake, excess raw foods, weak digestion (Qi deficiency).

Things that Treat Dampness:
Sweating, exercise, high vegetable diet (cooked), bitter, spicy, or pungent taste or smell, acupuncture, running cupping, gua sha, lymphatic drainage (endermologie™), Damp-resolving herbs.

湿热 Damp-Heat (*shī rè*)

When fluids congest in the cases of Phlegm-Damp, energy cannot flow freely and the body cannot rid itself of toxins. Over time this generates Heat. The combination of Dampness with Heat is very common in modern society and takes a long time of dedicated good behavior to treat. My teacher described clearing Damp-Heat from the body as being like separating flour from water. Dampness and Heat are two pathogens with opposite characteristics that come together to form a resilient glue. Damp is resolved by warming, drying, and aromatic treatments, all of which fuel Heat. While Heat is cleared by using cooling, moistening treatments, which exacerbate Dampness. Damp-Heat is a potential complication postpartum.

Signs of Damp-Heat:
Lethargy, purulent (pus-filled) discharges and infections, strong body odor, foul-smelling stools, excessive sweating, greasy scalp, yellow leucorrhea (vaginal discharge), red, itchy, fluid filled skin conditions (eczema, psoriasis), gallstones, liver disorders, bitter taste in the mouth.

> **KEY SIGNS OF DAMP-HEAT:**
>
> 1. Musty smell or strong body odor.
> 2. Thirst with no desire to drink.

Things that Cause Damp-Heat:
Longstanding Phlegm and Dampness in the body, longstanding digestive issues, stress, excessive alcohol (especially beer), excessive greasy and fatty foods, and excessive sugar intake.

Things that Treat Damp-Heat:
High vegetable diet, include more cooked foods to the degree Dampness predominates, increase raw foods and vegetable juices to the degree Heat predominates, bitter foods and drink, acupuncture, lymphatic drainage, running cupping, gua sha, Damp-Heat dispersing herbs.

燥 Dryness (*zào*)

The body is a wet system. Dryness is injurious particularly to the Lungs and Stomach. Dryness arises internally after Blood and body fluid loss (as occurs during and post-delivery), with Yin deficiency (hormonal depletion), and from exposure to environmental dryness (desert weather, airplane air).

Signs of Dryness:
Thinning skin, dryness (skin, eyes, vagina, hair), wrinkles, constipation.

Things that Cause Dryness:
Exposure to excessively dry environments, blood or body fluid loss, Blood and/or Yin deficiency, excessive cardio and sweating.

Things that Treat Dryness:
Cooling and moistening food and drink, soups, sipping water throughout the day, a little salty and sour taste, good fats, acupuncture, moistening herbs.

署 Summer-Heat (shǔ)

Summer-Heat is a pathological invasion that occurs from exposure to hot and damp weather during the summer months.

Signs of Summer-Heat:
Heat stroke, malaise, sensitivity to drafts, feeling hot, thirst, headache, and dark scanty urine.

Things that Cause Summer-Heat:
Hot and humid weather.

Things that Treat Summer-Heat:
Cooling, moistening foods, high vegetable diet, acupuncture, running cupping, Summer-Heat dispersing herbs.

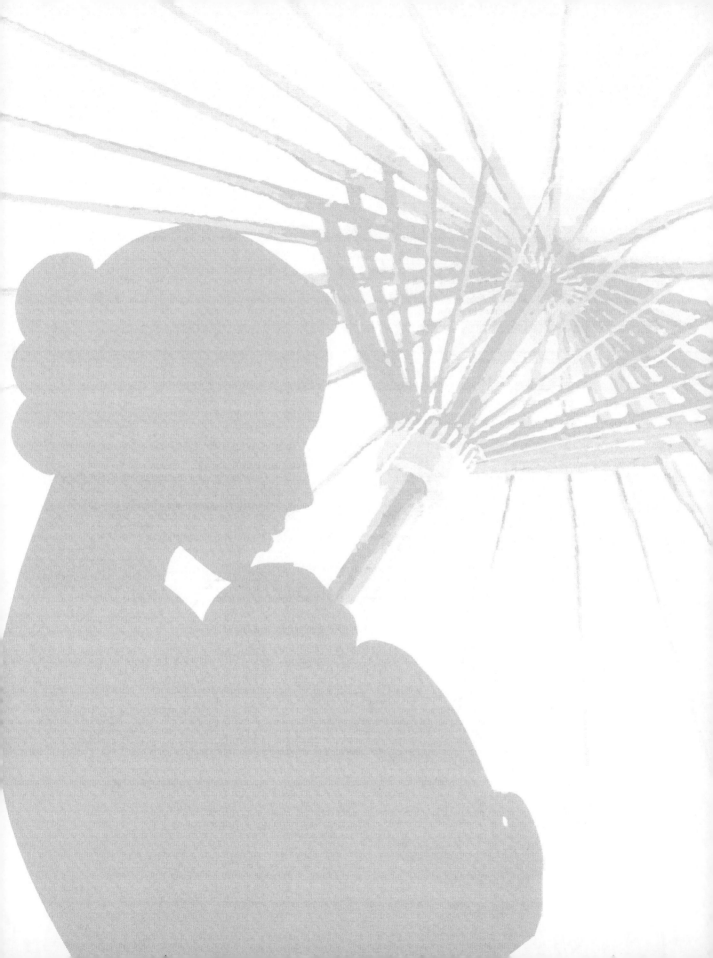

Chapter 3
Postpartum Traditions

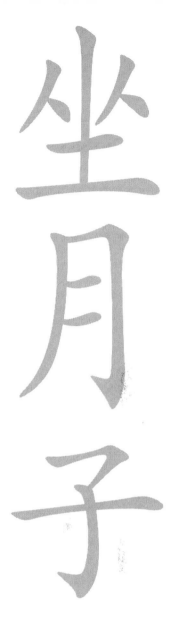

What is Postpartum Recovery?

Traditional Chinese culture was very clear about how women should spend their postpartum period as evidenced in their language. The term for puerperium in Mandarin Chinese is chǎn rù (产褥). Chǎn means "childbirth" and rù means "cotton-padded mattress." Postpartum Recovery is the English term for *zuò yuè zi* (坐月子), which literally means "sitting out the month (moon)." Postpartum recovery is a system of diet and lifestyle practices during the first 4-5 weeks after giving birth used to optimize a woman's recovery and long-term health after childbirth. The three key components are rest, diet, and a list of practices and restrictions.

Who Needs Postpartum Recovery?

Anyone who becomes pregnant needs the Postpartum Recovery Program™. Whether the fetus comes to term or not, whatever manner of birth, whatever age or condition of the mother, the woman must replenish herself after the nurturing she gave prenatally.

There is a saying in TCM gynecology that "miscarriage is more serious than childbirth".[1] It is more important to undergo postpartum recovery if you miscarry or have an abortion. In cases of abortion, miscarriage, C-section, mothers with weak constitutions, difficult birth, or mothers over 35, an extended postpartum recovery period is in order. This consists of 5 rather than 4 weeks. The reasoning is these cases are all more traumatic on women. In the cases of miscarriage or abortion, the natural cycle was interrupted, and the body will suffer for not having completed it. The other circumstances represent woman who have been weakened to a greater extent by giving birth. When in doubt, pamper yourself longer. Keep your reserves for when you need them. Ultimately trust your body to know when it is time to resume your normal level of activity. Use pregnancy and the time afterwards as a gift to remind yourself to listen to your body.

What Postpartum Recovery Promises

Postpartum recovery promises a means not only of regaining your pre-pregnancy physique, but to surpass it. It provides the means to renew yourself, look younger, heal constitutional weaknesses, and balance your hormones. Essentially it promises that your breasts will not sag, your body will not ache, and that your uterus and abdomen will return to normal size in record time.

Traditional culture insists that not following postpartum recovery guidelines leads women to obesity, body aches, cold hands and feet, hyperpigmentation (dark spots), wrinkles, loss of libido, premature aging, and gynecological disorders later on in life.

Women lose their heath and appearance after having children mainly due to ignorance, an injustice I seek to right with the information in this book. Modern Western culture has forgotten the concept of depletion, We value pushing through and doing more, ignoring the fact that a woman's body is robbed of reserves of vitality during pregnancy and childbirth.

---

1. Giovanni Maciocia. *Obstetrics & Gynecology in Chinese Medicine.* (Nanjing: Churchill Livingstone Press,1998), 60.

Modern Postpartum Practices

We have the advantage of crossing boundaries of culture and time to choose which practices best serve us during the postpartum month. Below are examples of postpartum care is addressed in modern Taiwan, France, and the U.S. to illustrate how modern medical systems can be set up to support women after childbirth.

Taiwan

Postpartum recovery is a part of Chinese and Taiwanese cultures, traditionally passed down from mother-in-law to new mother. Chinese postpartum recovery, or *zuò yuè zi* (坐月子), has been practiced at least as far back as the Song Dynasty (960-1279 AD). Early postpartum recovery was typically not pleasant for the new mom. She stayed at her mother-in-law's house at the mercy of her mother-in-law's interpretation of how postpartum care should be carried out. Ironically, a practice capable of empowering and uniting women was often used by powerless women to oppress each other, and the practice could be more akin to imprisonment than a vacation.

As postpartum practices are dying out in China, they have enjoyed a resurgence in the last 30 years in Taiwan. Independent and financially well-to-do Taiwanese women plan their own postpartum care. Women typically spend 7-10 days in the hospital after an uneventful birth after which they choose their postpartum care. They can choose to stay at postpartum birthing centers which are integrated with Western medicine to varying degrees. These provide luxury hotel-like accommodations for mother and family members, round-the-clock child care, prepared meals, assistance with postpartum practice, and often medical staff to monitor recovery and provide medical intervention as necessary. Integration with Western medicine has meant that certain traditional postpartum prohibitions have been done away with, such as the restriction on hair washing for the entire month.

A stay at a postpartum birthing centers is cost prohibitive for many moms. Less expensive options include simpler postpartum centers, meal delivery services, postpartum doulas, and babysitting services. You can find postpartum care centers in areas of the U.S. with large Chinese and Taiwanese immigrant populations.

France[2]

The French approach will seem extravagant to our Puritanical sensibilities. French health insurance covers integrative care methods such as homeopathy and wellness treatments are prescribed in special health spas for prenatal care and postpartum depression. Employed women have mandatory checkups each year that are fully covered by insurance.

---

2. This section is the author's synopsis of an interview by Veronica Anover with Dr. Stéphane Marmié, August 2013.

Physicians ask women what their plans are for children. The idea is to help women prepare 1 year ahead prior to getting pregnant. During this year of preparation women are supported in quitting addictions (particularly smoking), getting off the pill, and cleaning up their diet. Much like the TCM attitude, women are encouraged to be in an optimal state of health when they conceive to increase the chances of a healthy pregnancy for both mother and fetus. Prenatal care begins with conception.

After a woman conceives, medical care follows the same protocol as it does in the U.S. in terms of checkups, ultrasound, genetic tests, etc., only it is completely covered by insurance,

During delivery, emphasis is on massaging and relaxing the perineum. Part of protecting women against vaginal tears is also keeping a woman's diet healthy and her weight within normal range. French women are recommended a maximum weight gain of 10-12 kilos (22-26 pounds), slightly lower than here. The difference is that in France the physician monitors and advises his/her patient on this matter throughout the pregnancy. Physicians are strict on diet (in a French way), no ice cream or processed food, while foods like leafy greens, fish, liver, and of course cheese are encouraged. Smoking is strictly discouraged, but women are allowed up to 1 cup of coffee and 1 glass of wine per day.

Insufficient weight gain in the mother leads to nutritional impairments in the mother and potential developmental issues in the fetus. Excessive weight gain increases complications such as gestational diabetes and preeclampsia. It also creates bigger babies which mean greater risk of vaginal tears, episiotomies, and C-sections.

Delivery options are similar to the U.S. Doulas, midwives, and home births are all available, only home births are unpopular.

Postpartum

A woman who has a vaginal birth without complications stays in the hospital 2-4 days after delivery. A lactation consultant goes to the new mother's house and makes sure that breast feeding is going well. A kinesiologist also visits the new mother and gives her exercises to rebuild her abdomen and pelvic floor as part of the rééducation périnéale. All of this is covered by insurance. Daycare is free and new moms receive one year of free nanny services. There is one year of maternity leave and also paternity leave. Postpartum depression still happens. Women are treated integratively, with medications, thermal spas, and other treatments.

OBGYNs check on healing of the abdomen, inquire on exercise, and monitor women's weight to make sure the body is bouncing back. The expectation is that women will get their body and identity back in about three months' time, and the medical establishment supports women in this process. Breastfeeding is encouraged for four months to one year. Dr. Stéphane Marmié feels that the longer periods of lactation are advised as a safeguard to deficient nutrition being given in the home. He feels that at least four months is ideal, and more than this is optional as long as there are good food options.

United States

In the U.S. women typically spend two days in the hospital after an uneventful vaginal delivery. Many women are grateful to be out of there quickly to avoid disease and negligence.

What the government provides in France, American women must rely on the kindness of others. Recent years have seen a rise in communities of women who help each other during postpartum and later. Beyond this we need to realize as a culture how critical it is for a woman and her newborn's health to receive care and support at this time. Physicians in the U.S. also need to support women in this process, as the postpartum period is a time many women injure their health, though the litigious nature of our culture will likely impede this.

We place a high value on self-reliance, which taken to the extreme is unhealthy. There are times when we are meant to lean on others and receive support. Networks are helpful, but may not reach those most in need. Systems decide how the weak and vulnerable end up. The program in the next section offers steps you can take as an individual to ensure you have an optimum postpartum recovery. My hope is that it will inspire changes in postpartum care for all women.

The
Postpartum Recovery
Program™

Postpartum Recovery Plan™ Guide

Prohibitions

1. Avoid drafts and cold temperature for 4-5 weeks (page 70).
2. Avoid cold food and drinks for 4-5 weeks (page 68).
3. Do not walk around with wet hair for 4-5 weeks (page 68).
4. No tub bathing for 4-5 weeks (page 69).
5. Do not carry your baby or nurse sitting up for 4-5 weeks (page 87).
6. Do not lift weight for 4-5 weeks (page 86).
7. Do not go up and down stairs for 4-5 weeks (page 86).
8. Avoid sexual intercourse for 6 weeks (page 107).
9. Do not overeat for 4-5 weeks.

Practices

1. Get support (page 64).
2. Keep warm (page 70).
3. Stay home (page 64).
4. Sleep for 10 hours a night and rest (page 64).
5. Wear a postpartum girdle 1-3 months (page 82).
6. Protect your eyes (page 66).
7. Protect your vagina and perineum (page 100).
8. Strengthen your core, when cleared by your doctor(page 89).
9. Perform pelvic floor rehabilitation exercises daily (page 75).

Diet

1. Eat a high protein diet (page 120).
2. Eat mostly cooked foods.
3. Take placenta capsules daily, if you choose (page 122).
4. Drink Red Date Tea for the first week to cleanse the Liver (page 157).

Preparation Checklist

Organizing Support

1. Who will do the housekeeping (laundry, vacuuming, washing dishes, etc.)?
2. Who will carry and care for the baby?
3. Who will feed the baby at night?
4. Who will prepare your meals? Or will you prepare them ahead of time and freeze them?

Supplies

1. Postpartum girdle.
2. Teas and medicinals.
3. Key ingredients.

Chart of Recovery Milestones

1. Lochia passes during first 2 -4 weeks. If lochia is still present after 4 weeks it can indicate an infection.
2. Menses returns at 4 months. If menstruation does not return it is a sign of Blood deficiency or hormonal imbalance.
3. Good mood, sleep, and steady return of libido over first 3 months.
4. Gradual recovery of abdomen and pelvic floor over first 3 months.

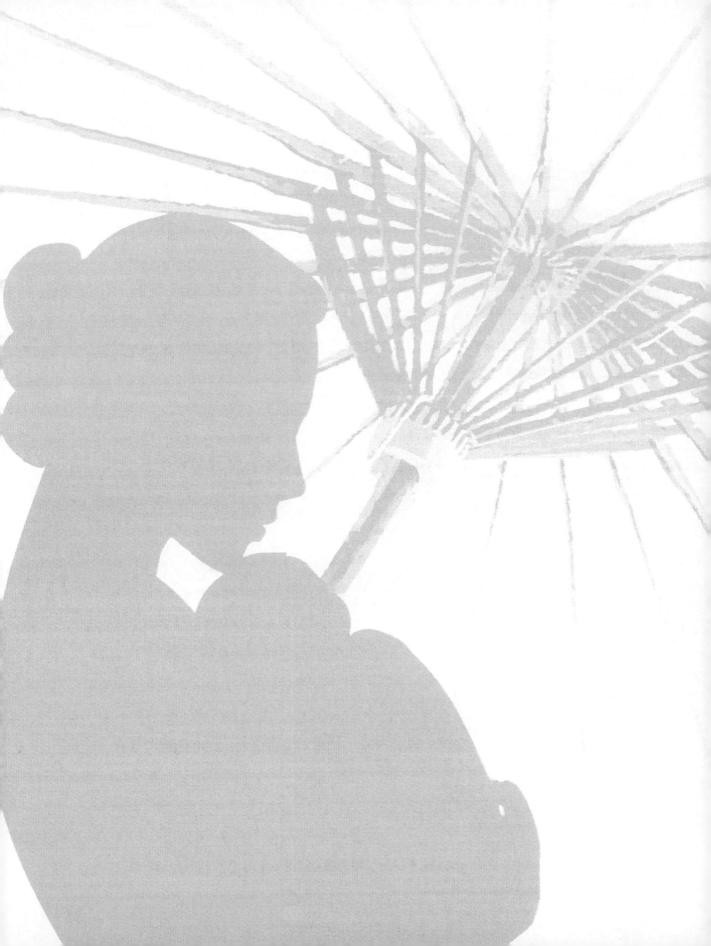

Chapter 4
Practices &
Restrictions

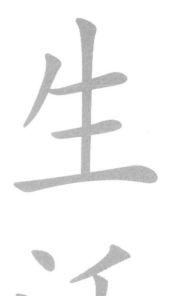
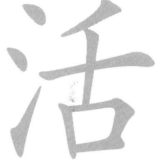

The lifestyle practices in this section comprise the first half of the Postpartum Recovery Program™. Diet constitutes the second half and will be covered in the next section on postpartum diet. What you read in these pages will likely seem extreme. If you are like most modern women you have been conditioned to ignore your body's natural rythms, particularly the need for rest and nurturing. Use this time to reconnect with yourself and develop a deeper bond with your baby.

During the first month after birth stay home and get ample rest. Be sure to keep warm. This protects your fragile immune system and speeds restoration of your body and mind. Resist the urge to jump back into your normal schedule. Doing too much too quickly will set you back in your recovery and leave you prone to premature aging, hormonal imbalance, depression, poor milk supply, organ prolapse, poor wound healing, infection, and other issues.

The Third Trimester & Delivery

Though pregnancy and delivery are beyond the scope of this book, I wanted to include some tips that have helped my patients. The birthing process and bringing forth of new life has long been held over women as a curse of pain; some even citing it as retribution for Eve's behavior in the Garden of Eden. It is time to let go of this paradigm of fear. Yes, birth is a rite of passage. Let it be a passage in which we support one another and one in which we make our own choices. We have choice now to transform old constructs and to, as master yoga instructor Flossie Park says, "Be not what is expected of us, but what is true of us."

Protecting Your Belly

Beginning the third or fourth month of pregnancy, keep the abdomen moisturized by applying organic coco butter, shea butter, avocado oil, jojoba oil, coconut oil, and/or some other super-moisturizing oils to prevent stretch marks (I use 302 Body Massage Oil at Cinnabar Clinic). During last trimester wear a belly band to protect the abdomen, pelvic floor, and low back.

> **SECRET TO A BEAUTIFUL BELLY**
>
> Andrea was a stunning Columbian woman. When she lifted her shirt to show me her post-pregnancy belly there was not a single mark. Her secret was *aceite de germen de trigo* (wheatgerm oil), which is a thick oil high in vitamin E and a long tradition in treating scars. She applied it 2-3 times a day as soon as her belly began to show in her fourth month or so. After applying the oil she would put on a loose band around her abdomen to seal in the oil and protect her clothes. She continued through her postpartum month, though she was less diligent after the baby was born.

Preparing Your Pelvic Floor

Practice both strengthening and increasing the stretching ability of your pelvic floor and vaginal opening if you are preparing for vaginal delivery. Strengthening the pelvic floor will help you to hold up the fetus while pregnant, pushing during delivery, and recovering after (see exercises on page 76). It is also important to learn to relax your pelvic floor fully to ease birth and discourage tearing.

Tearing occurs in between 44-79% of births.[1],[2] Perineal massage is a practice whereby the mother-to-be, or her partner, massages the skin between the vagina and anus (the perineum) daily, beginning at week 34. To do this, place your (or your partner's) thumbs shallowly into your vagina (no more than an inch or so) and press the perineal floor down towards the bowel and to both sides until you feel a slight stretching sensation. Maintain the pressure for about a minute before resting. Alternately, you can use an Epi-No™ birthing trainer which is a balloon-like device you insert into

1. Birth. 2005 Sep;32(3):164-9. Maternal position at midwife-attended birth and perineal trauma: is there an association? Retrieved from www.ncbi.nlm.nih.gov/pubmed?term=16128969

2. Birth. 2007 Dec;34(4):282-90. Perineal outcomes and maternal comfort related to the application of perineal warm packs in the second stage of labor: a randomized controlled trial. Retrieved from www.ncbi.nlm.nih.gov/pubmed/18021143

the vagina and inflate to stretch the perineum.[3] A midwife, doctor, or doula can also massage the perineum and use hot compresses during birth to prevent tearing and speed delivery.

I recommend reading up on the episiotomy[4] debate so you can decide ahead of time if you want to do an episiotomy or reserve it for emergencies. You will want to discuss this with your physician, midwife, doula, etc. as part of your birth plan. One of my teachers, Dr. Jiang Zheng, recommended that vaginal delivery was better for women under 35, and C-section for women over 35. The pelvic floor tends to become loose as we age. Thus the ability for the vagina to bounce after birth may not be as strong.

Visualizing Your Birth

Flossie Park recommends getting into a squatting position and visualizing your birth. It is a great way to infuse associations of relaxation, ease, and familiarity into muscle memory. Squatting positions the birth canal at its shortest, while lying down with the feet up places the birth canal at its longest.

Tuning Into Your Breath

Qigong, prenatal yoga, and meditation classes are all great places to practice tuning into your own breath. Birthing coaches and hypnotherapists will also likely discuss breathing techniques. The breath is your connection to the unconscious, subtle operations going on in your body. It is why controlling the breath is used as a technique for pain relief, meditation, and increased athletic performance.

Finding Your Voice

I have heard stories from numerous women who were shushed or shamed into being quiet during labor. One nurse even told me that some women "can be so dramatic" and yell "to get attention." With this attitude it is no wonder that some women consider home birth a better option. Birth is about following your inner guidance.

One of the most powerful ways we move energy is to vocalize and we do this naturally. In karate class they teach you to yell when you strike. Weightlifters yell and grunt when they move heavy weight. Why then should you not make noise when you are delivering a baby? We as women have largely been socialized to hold our tongues, to keep our voices high rather than speaking from our bellies, and to speak softly lest we disturb someone. If you are to get into your body and into your power you must use your voice. Practice saying mantras or singing loudly. Liberate your voice,

---

3. Available at www.epi-no.com.au

4. An episiotomy is an incision made into the perineum to prevent tearing during delivery. Episiotomies are necessary when a worse tear is imminent. The debate is on whether elective incisions are easier to suture, cause less damage than natural tears, and preserve vaginal tightness better.

PREGNANCY AND MOTHERHOOD AS SACRED OPPORTUNITY

An interview with Flossie Park, a wise yoga instructor and teacher (interview with the author, July 20, 2013).

"We need to bring back our concept of rituals. We have lost our rituals. There is a huge rite of passage as women become mothers."

Preparing for Delivery:

"Prenatal yoga helps the body to be strong and in alignment to prepare for birth. Also, during delivery we use the same side of the brain as we do in Yin Yoga [an internalized style of yoga]. We need to get used to being in that side of the brain. This also helps the baby's development. The baby's brain develops according to the mother's emotions. They either develop fight or flight or develop their creative brain.

We need to get connected with our breath and our bodies. Learn to listen to your breath the way you will listen to your baby's breath. Connect with your voice and the 5th chakra. Birth is very vocal. Practice exercising your voice. I see most women giving away their power to doctors or to their mothers."

On Delivery:

"All our fears are learned. Fears about birth and being a mom are learned. Every fear you have ever held was taught to you. I don't believe we are meant to suffer. We suffer when we are in separation consciousness. With birth and delivery we have bought into the story. We have to know how to listen to our bodies. So don't resist the pain. Instead, find the animal part of yourself. Get out of your head and into your body.

Most women don't trust their bodies. They don't need to read all this information. Your body knows how to give birth. What you have to do is trust your body. The body is so sacred. Sit in awe of how the body pulls itself back together so fast. You need to take care of yourself."

On Postpartum:

"After delivery there is no yoga for at least 6 weeks. Prenatal yoga is very gentle as blood pressure and volume are higher. This is not the time to stay in shape. For women with this attitude it will be difficult after birth. The postpartum period is really about honoring this body. It is an expression of the divine. What is the attitude towards the body? [During postpartum] do something for yourself. Don't do something out of obligation, do it out of inspiration. It is not just about getting your body back.

I am a proponent of the Divine Feminine. The Divine Feminine is Wisdom, Love, and Power. All a woman can do [postpartum] is nurse the baby. She is so in her power as a woman and as a mother. And yet there is this message that she is not valuable just being a mother; not contributing."

On Parenting:

"All a baby needs is your love and to know they are valued. Babies need nature, not overstimulation. Put them in nature and they remember their divinity. Put them in a play pen with a bunch of gadgets and they learn sensory overload.

Another important point is the baby has to come through you, and not for you. Trust your intuition; be in touch with feelings; trust yourself that you know how to parent.

When we get into stillness, humanness and spirit unite in the heart."

otherwise you will be missing out on a powerful tool. Find an advocate during your delivery who will support your full expression. If they do not, do not invite them to your delivery.

Let Go of Outcome

This is the hardest one, but it is the lesson life gives us most. You can prepare everything perfectly and sometimes it just turns out differently. Do not blame yourself. You may also change your mind. Women have different levels of pain tolerance, and also different levels of pain. Exhaustion will erode your ability to deal with pain. If you need pain killers, take them.

Rest

The postpartum month is a lesson in being, not doing.

Purpose: strengthen the body, protect against pathogens.

Do Not Leave the House

Do not go on excursions, grocery shopping, etc. Do not spend time outside unless it is a nice warm 77-82° F with no wind. You are protecting yourself from getting tired and also from coming in contact with potential illnesses.

Rest Requirements

Rest as much as possible for the entire Postpartum Recovery Program™. Of all the recommendations, this is the single most important and hardest one for new mothers to comply with. The first two weeks spend as much time sleeping as you can bear. Pump your breast milk and get 10 hours of real sleep a night. After two weeks you can increase activity around the house. However, never let yourself get tired the first month. This admonition is for the newborn as well. He/she should be allowed to rest as much as possible. When mother and baby emerge into the world at the end of the first month they will do so strong and ready.

Communal Assistance

The only way you will get rest during the first month is to organize help. Some women will be lucky enough to recruit from family and friends. If this is not an option, hire doulas, nannies, and housekeepers to keep the household running, meals prepared, and the baby cared for at night. As much as possible, surround yourself with loving, supportive people. You want to find a community of people who not only help, but who remind you of what is important.

A key feature of postpartum recovery and its variants in various cultures is its dependence on family and friends. Your partner should take the month off to oversee care. Extended family and/or friends take turns running household chores and caring for the newborn. Not only does this allow for the greatest care of mother and baby, it places importance on bonding the new baby to the community.

If You Can Not Get Help

If you do not have family and friends who can help out and you cannot afford to hire help, organize your postpartum as best you can.

1. **Set your priorities.** The most important thing is for you and your baby to be rested and

---

KALI'S STORY – HOW A YOUNG, SINGLE MOM GOT HER REST

Kali had always been a positive, happy, optimistic person, and came to my clinic when she began feeling down and felt unable to shake it. She bounced back quickly and we were all excited when she came in with the news that she was pregnant; a child she deeply wanted.

Kali had developed friendships in her time in San Diego, but her deepest friendships and close family were all in Northern California. Her boyfriend, though she loved him, was still immature and overwhelmed with the impending responsibility. Thus he was not able to be there for her in the way Kali and her daughter deserved. But then, challenging situations often hide blessings. When Kali walked into our clinic after her delivery, she carried in the most mellow, glowing baby. What was her secret?

Firstly, Kali exuded a calm, grounded, loving energy that her daughter, Niyah, no doubt responded to. Secondly, she really wanted her baby. I have observed no greater strength than in a determined mother. Thirdly, Kali slept with her baby. This way she was able to nurse Niyah at night without disturbing her own sleep as much.

But the real trick was what Kali called the "baby spa," a ritual she learned from Jamaica Moon, whose mother, Lisa was a midwife (before she passed in 2006). Lisa Moon called the baby spa the key to life.[1]

The baby spa includes playing relaxing music or singing to your baby while massaging them with oil. You talk to your baby about their body as you massage each body part. Then you bathe in the tub with your baby. Moon claimed the baby spa teaches confidence and independence from their mother especially in the early days as they still feel they are part of us. This daily ritual helps the baby develop physically and emotionally.

After the baby spa ritual, Kali would bundle up Niyah and leave her resting while Kali would warm up dinner. This ritual was nurturing for both mother and baby. It gave Niyah what all babies (and living things) need: undivided attention and connection. It also gave Kali what she needed: a baby habituated to settling down and sleeping at night.

---

1. A video of Lisa Moon can be found here: www.youtu.be/4_RTEx-VuYw

---

fed. Your newborn also needs focused attention and connection. Everything else is a far second. Give up on the idea of having a well-kept house or entertaining visitors.

2. **Co-Sleeping.** If you do not have help at night the best way to get sleep is to have your baby close to you. This way you do not have to get out of bed and fully wake up to nurse. For descriptions of safe co-sleeping practices I recommend Dr. Sears' books.[5]

3. **Freeze Your Meals.** If you do not have anyone to prepare your meals, prepare a month's worth ahead of time. Prepare your meals and divide them into meal-size portions. You may have to buy a small freezer. Do not assume you will have time and energy to prepare

---

5. William Sears, Martha Sears, James Sears, and Robert Sears. *The Baby Sleep Book: The Complete Guide to a Good Night's Rest for the Whole Family.* (Little Brown, 2005).
William Sears, Martha Sears, James Sears, Robert Sears. *The Baby Book: Everything You Need to Know About Your Baby From Birth to Age Two.* (Little Brown, Revised Edition, 2013).
William Sears. *SIDS: A Parent's Guide to Understanding and Preventing Sudden Infant Death Syndrome* (Little Brown, 1995).

regular healthy meals for yourself after delivery. You can also prepare packets of congee (page 162) that you can add to a rice cooker or crock pot and just add water and cook.

4. **Multiple Children.** If you already have children, you will need to find support for the existing children. It is entirely too much for a woman to recover from childbirth, nurture a newborn, while running a household and care for existing children. This is when most women crash. If you are in this predicament do the best you can and be kind to yourself.

Keep Calm – Avoid Stress

When we are Qi and Blood deficient, as women are after delivery, we are more easily and deeply hurt by painful events. Take extra care to ensure you are surrounded by loving, supportive people (this is a good life strategy in general). Your helpers should buffer stress and challenges from you for the 30-40 days. Also, listen to relaxing music.

Do Not Shed Tears

There is a Chinese saying that "One teardrop from a postpartum woman is as valuable as 500g of gold." Postpartum, the body fluids are depleted and should be conserved as much as possible.

Protect Your Eyes - Minimize TV and Reading

The eyes are dependent on healthy Liver Blood and Kidney Yin to function, both of which are deficient at this time. Watch TV or read for shorter stretches at a time, taking a break every 15 minutes or so to prevent eye strain. Make sure to massage your eyes daily.

Eye Massage Techniques:

1. Use a warm wet towel compress on your eyes to begin.
2. Close your eyes. Use your thumb or middle fingers to press firmly working your way around the orbital bone.
3. Use your thumb knuckles to do a figure 8 pattern around your eyes.
4. Use both middle fingers to press from the center of the hairline out, working down to the temples.

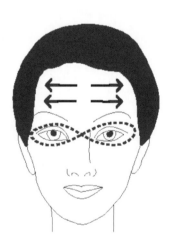

Figure 4.1. Eye Massage

Simplify Meditation & Spiritual Practice

If you had a meditation or spiritual practice prior to giving birth, you will have to amend it during this time. When the body is weak it is harder to focus and put out the mental energy. Prayer and meditation take energy. Instead, practice simple presence. Take the opportunity to connect with your newborn, and to focus on your heart and loving energy when you remember to.

Practice Self-Forgiveness

A postpartum woman's proud husband posted on social media a long post on how brave his wife was, and called her a "superwoman" for having had a completely natural birth. This man meant no harm and was no doubt supporting his wife, and yet it demonstrates a phenomenon in our culture in which birth and child-rearing have become another arena in which to judge and compete. Women who "fail" at natural childbirth and breastfeeding are somehow less than women who do. Women, either by nature or conditioning, are already hard on themselves. When a new life is involved, added to every misstep comes the guilt that we have ruined our child's chances for a healthy future.

Babies need to feel they are wanted and loved. They need to eat frequently, get plenty of physical affection, and be kept clean. If you cover these consistently it is okay if you say or do something imperfectly on occasion. Sometimes things are beyond your control, like if there is a complication during delivery or your baby is unable to latch. Babies do not need expensive devices and toys. They need connection with kind people, stimulation to their language, physical movement, and creativity, and to experience nature.

Keeping Warm

Purpose: strengthen the body, protect against pathogens, and promote discharge of lochia.[6]

The prohibitions are strictest during the first 2 weeks when the body is weakest and the lochia is discharging, and slacken somewhat the 3rd and 4th weeks when the body has regained some strength.

Avoid Cold Water

Avoid drinking or washing with cold water. Cold water internally is taxing on Stomach Qi and puts out digestive fire, interrupting digestion. Cold water externally can easily cause Cold invasion, leading to chronic joint pain and stagnating blood in the uterus.

Do Not Walk Around With Wet Hair

Wash your hair less frequently, wash it with warm water in a warm bathroom, and thoroughly dry it with a hairdryer. Never walk around with wet hair even if it is summertime. After giving birth the pores are lax and susceptible to Cold invasion (i.e. colds and joint pain). Cold invasion in the scalp can lead to stagnation and blood congealing in the uterus.

In traditional Chinese postpartum care, women did not wash their hair for the entire month. Instead they used the Alcohol Wash Method.[7] To follow this, make a mixture of equal parts 95% isopropyl rubbing alcohol and warm water. Add a few drops of essential oils for fragrance and antibacterial qualities.[8] Use a comb to part the hair and use a cotton ball to apply

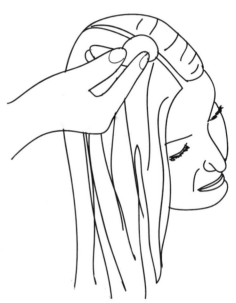

Figure 4.2. Alcohol Wash Method

the alcohol and warm water mixture. Cover the entire scalp. Comb the hair afterwards. Be sure to thoroughly wash the comb with soap and water after each use. Use the Alcohol Wash method daily,

---

6. Lochia is the normal vaginal discharge after birth made up of blood, mucus, and placental tissue. It is important that these materials be discharged and the uterus be clean in order to avoid long-term gynecological problems. During C-section the uterus should be cleansed of these to speed healing.

7. Shuqi Zhuang. *Postpartum Recovery Program; a Manual of Rules and Recipes for the Postpartum Woman.* (Taiwan: Guang He Chu Ban She, 2005). ISBN 9578807015

8. Citrus and rosemary essential oils help to cut oiliness. Clove, cinnamon, and other spice essential oils are antibacterial.

PROTECTING & BLESSING YOUR BABY

Newborns must acclimate to a dense, scary world compared to where they came from. We should make this transition as gentle as possile. This adjustment is not just emotional, it is also physical. Until children reach 6 years of age their Spleens are not fully developed. This means their immune and digestive systems are fragile. This also means that small children are unable to protect themselves from negative energy in the same way adults can. Traditional cultures have rituals to protect newborns spiritually as well as physically. Protecting your baby and blessing him or her can be done in the context of any religion or independent of religion. **Note:** any time you use an herbal tincture or essential oil on a baby (or animal) for blessing or protection purposes, first place some on your finger and wipe it off on your clothes or a cloth. Then touch your baby. Their skin and senses are very sensitive. Always dilute essential oils in a carrier oil before applying them on anyone.

Keeping Your Baby Close - will keep your baby safe within your energetic field or that of other loving adults.

Goldenseal - is a gentle yet powerful plant to clear all manner of negative energy.[1] Since you are using the Qi of the plant, all you need is a few drops of tincture to clear a space. Sprinkle some around the crib and any openings (windows and doors) at night. Also touch your fingers with goldenseal to the baby's forehead, heart, and belly. Do all of this while visualizing angelic, protective, healing energy around your baby.[2]

Sage - is a popular choice for smudging. It has a grandmotherly energy that sorts out energy that does not belong and escorts it out.[3] If there is an argument or emotional disturbance, open the windows and light a sage bundle to clear the air afterwards.

---

1. Poppy Mehlhaff. "Animal Healing". (lecture, San Diego, April 27, 2014). Poppy Mehlhaff is an expert in the field of animal healing and communication.

2. Be sure to buy organically grown goldenseal. Avoid wildcrafted sources. Wild goldenseal has been over-harvested to near extinction.

3. It is interesting to note that the physical effects of plants in medicine mirror their energetic function in plant spirit medicine.

---

prior to one of your meals. Some women may prefer to braid their hair during this time. Alcohol is used as it astringes the pores.[9]

Bathing Restrictions

Do not soak in a tub for the entire postpartum month to avoid introducing pathogens into the vagina and uterus. Take shorter, warm showers in a warm bathroom. Make sure to dry yourself thoroughly and do not leave the bathroom until your pores have returned to normal.

In traditional Chinese postpartum care, women do not bathe normally for the first two weeks

---

9. The use of alcohol as a washing method seems at first peculiar. There is, however, a tradition in the West of alcohol used to astringe the pores on the skin and guard against Wind invasion. Famed American strongman Adolph Nordequest writing in 1905, made suggestions on how to safely take care of one's self after exercising and inducing perspiration. After using a dry towel to dry off completely, he advised readers to apply a solution of 95% alcohol, witch hazel, and arnica, which "not only [will] have the effect of closing the pores, but it will relieve sore muscles." Viking. Strength and Health; How Disease May be Successfully Combated by Physical Culture. (New York: Richard K. Fox, 1905), 27. Accessed from www.Sandowplus.co.uk

postpartum. Instead they use the sponge bath method below. At the beginning of the third week they resume showering. The reasoning is the pores are lax postpartum and highly susceptible to Wind invasion.

Sponge Bath Method: Mix warm water and rice wine in equal parts. Add 1 tbsp 95% isopropyl rubbing alcohol and one tbsp. of salt. Mix. Use a hand towel or sponge dipped in the mixture to wash yourself. For the genitals, use a strong green tea decoction, with salt and rubbing alcohol. The teeth and face can be washed normally, only be sure to use warm water. After washing yourself apply talcum powder to your abdomen before refastening the binding or postpartum girdle.[10]

Maintain a Warm Ambient Temperature

Maintain an ambient temperature of 77-82° F (25-28° C) at all times, no matter what the season. Block or redirect air conditioning vents from blowing on you. Wear long pants, long sleeves, a scarf, and socks at all times. Cover up as needed. Do not allow yourself to feel cold.

Warm the Abdomen

Your acupuncturist may use moxa (or moxibustion) if your abdomen feels cold to the touch and/or there is abdominal pain. Moxa is an important modality in TCM where ai ye (mugwort) is dried, then burned indirectly over areas with impeded circulation. The plant's oils enter the

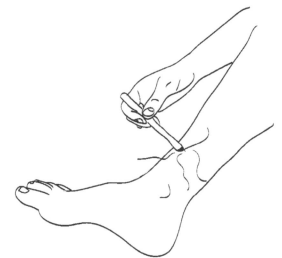

Figure 4.3. Moxibustion of the lower leg

body through the smoke, warming the channels and moving the blood. This makes moxa an ideal treatment during postpartum recovery. Your acupuncturist may also instruct you how to use a moxa stick on the lower abdomen, low back, and along the inner shins (Figure 4.3) at home. Typically, patients are instructed to use a swirling or pecking motion until the area feels warmed.

---

10. The concept of the sponge bath is common to all postpartum recovery traditions in China. This washing solution recipe was taken from Shuqi Zhuang. Postpartum Recovery Program; a Manual of Rules and Recipes for the Postpartum Woman. (Taiwan: Guang He Chu Ban She, 2005). ISBN 9578807015

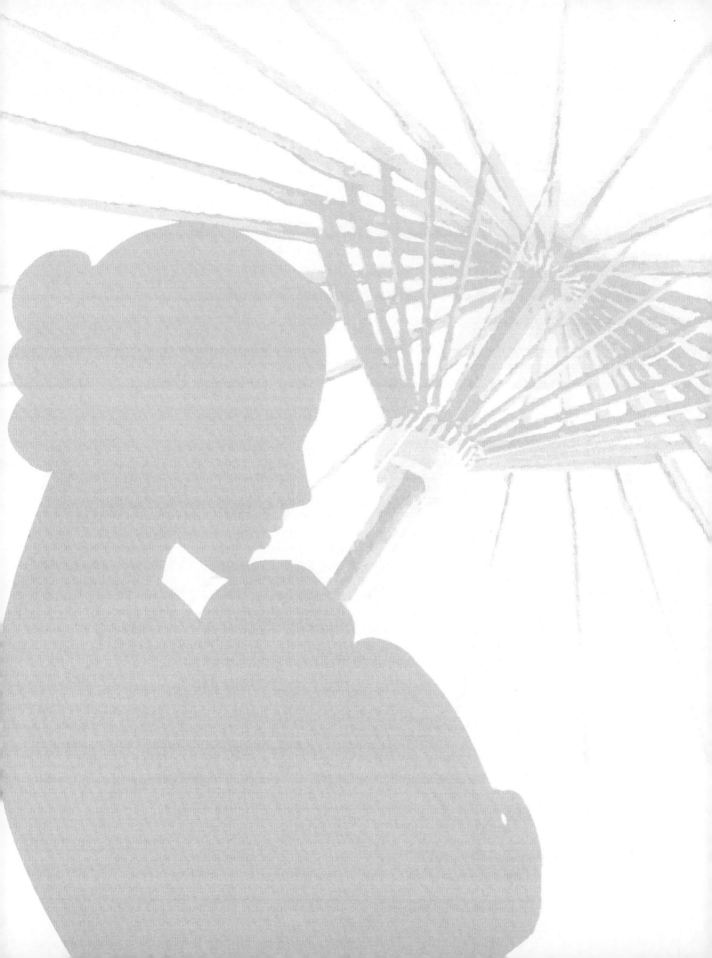

Chapter 5

Rehabilitating the Pelvic Floor 盆底

Many of the postpartum practices and restrictions are to protect and recover the pelvic floor and abdominal cavity after delivery. This focus on the pelvic floor may seem excessive if you have never experienced a problem, but pelvic floor strength is key to increasing general strength and to improving how a woman ages. Ancient Daoists dedicated a huge part of their practice to strengthening the pelvic floor, which they associated with conserving Jing. A strong pelvic floor keeps our vital energy (and organs and bodily fluids) from leaking out.

Our pelvic floor is involved in many of our daily activities. When we lift something heavy our abdominal muscles get involved. Strong contraction of the abdominal muscles puts a great deal of downward pressure on the pelvic floor. When the pelvic floor is strong and engaged, there will be equal force pressing up, increasing our ability to lift. However, when these muscles are weak, they cannot withstand the downward pressure and there is a high likelihood of organ prolapse. When we sneeze or cough, it also contracts the abdomen putting downward pressure on the pelvic floor. If this area is weak, it can cause urinary or fecal incontinence.

The pelvic floor is a canopy of muscles and ligaments. It is the only thing holding our internal organs up in our body. Pregnancy puts a great deal of pressure on the pelvic floor and abdominal muscles, even prior to delivery. Diastasis recti is a common condition in which the rectus abdominis actually tears (more on page 90). The pelvic floor is further weakened during vaginal delivery. In order to repair the pelvic floor and abdominal wall, all women should follow this three-point approach after giving birth: 1) wear a postpartum girdle, 2) avoid lifting, and 3) practice daily pelvic floor exercises. (The postpartum girdle and restrictions on lifting are covered in the next chapter on abdominal recovery).

Benefits of These Practices
- Avoid organ prolapse
- Regain connection with abdomen and pelvic floor
- Support thorough healing of the abdomen
- Avoid issues with urinary or fecal incontinence
- Regain your waistline and flat belly

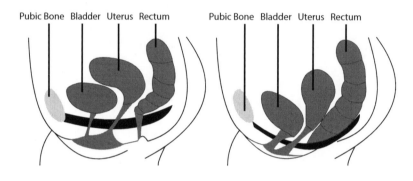

Figure 5.1. Organ Prolapse

Pelvic Floor Exercises

Resist the urge to quickly get your toned abdominals back. You first have to build up your pelvic floor and assist your abdominal cavity in shrinking back to normal size (aided by a postpartum girdle, nutrition, and herbs).

It is difficult to give exact time frames for beginning these exercises. It depends on if you had vaginal tears, a C-section, or a relatively easy delivery and how quickly you are healing. Most women can start activating their pelvic floor the day after delivery.

Pelvic floor muscles are synonymous with the PC or Pubococcygeus muscle. The PC muscle originates in the pubic bone and inserts at the base of the coccyx, forming the pelvic floor. It controls contraction and relaxation of the urethra (urine flow), vagina (during orgasm and childbirth), and anus (helps avoid hemorrhoids). The PC muscle holds the weight of our internal organs. Pelvic floor exercises are also known as Kegels, named after Dr. Kegel, a proponent of them.

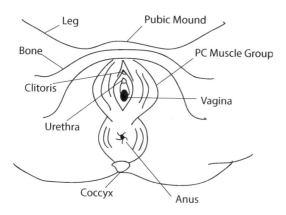

Leg
Pubic Mound
Bone
PC Muscle Group
Clitoris
Vagina
Urethra
Coccyx
Anus

Figure 5.2. Pubococcygeus (PC) Muscle

Pelvic Floor Exercises

For the postpartum month, practice most of your exercises lying down. This makes use of gravity to help lift the pelvic floor. Short daily practice is preferred to longer sporadic practice. Choose one or two exercises at a time. After the postpartum month you can progress to using a jade egg, or other vaginal strengthening tool, and adding weighted resistance.

Finding Your Pelvic Floor Muscles

The easiest way to find the pelvic floor muscles is to practice stopping urination and then allowing it to flow. Once you have found your muscles, imagine pulling up as you squeeze. Then practice increasing the tension. Next you can progress to the exercises. After childbirth you may feel numbness, pain, or an inability to connect to your pelvic floor muscles. If this is the case, imagine controlling these muscles when performing the exercises. Eventually this will turn into actual control.

Practices

Perform these exercises every time you put on your postpartum girdle; i.e. after every meal and after you bathe. This ensures that you will be getting several repetitions in daily and you have another activity to remind you.

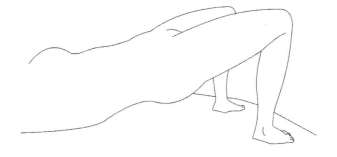

Figure 5.3. Bridge Pose

Exercise 5.1. Basic Bridge Kegels

1. Put on your girdle to protect your back.
2. Lie face up in a mini-bridge position. Press into the ground with your heels and squeeze your knees towards each other activating the inner thighs and pelvic floor.
3. Tense your pelvic floor and imagine pulling it up as high as you can towards your head. Hold for a count of 5.
4. Bring hips down and fully relax your body. A fully functioning muscle can perform the full range from strong tension to complete relaxation. This is what gives a muscle elasticity.
5. Resume the mini-bridge position. This time try to tense the pelvic floor without engaging your legs and buttocks. Tense your pelvic floor and pull it up. Hold for a count of 5.

6. Fully relax.
7. Repeat for 10-20 repetitions. When you have worked up to 20 repetitions you are ready to progress to the Intermediate Bridge Kegels below.

Exercise 5.2. Intermediate Bridge Kegels

1. If you feel strong enough, practice this exercise before putting on your girdle.
2. Lie face up in a mini-bridge position. Press into the ground with your heels and squeeze your knees towards each other activating the inner thighs and pelvic floor.
3. Tense your pelvic floor and imagine pulling it up as high as you can towards your head. Hold the contraction for a count of 3 then add 3 rapid contractions.
4. Bring hips down and fully relax your body.
5. Resume the mini-bridge position. Using increased tension pulling up higher, tense your pelvic floor and pull it up. Hold for a count of 3 then add 3 rapid contractions.
6. Fully relax.
7. Repeat for 10-20 repetitions. When you have worked up to 20 repetitions you are ready to progress to the advanced exercises below.

Exercise 5.3. Horizontal Isolation

After you have mastered controlling the pelvic floor as a unit, begin to isolate three zones: the clitoris, the vagina, and the anus. This will seem impossible at first. Focus your attention on each zone and imagine that you are tensing and relaxing only that zone while keeping the others relaxed. Over time imagination will turn into actual muscle control.

1. Lie face up with your legs extended and arms at your sides.
2. Fully relax your pelvic floor.
3. Imagine tightening the muscles around your clitoris and pulling it up. Hold for a count of 5.
4. Relax.
5. Repeat 10 times.
6. Imagine tightening the muscles around your vagina and pulling it up. Hold for a count of 5.
7. Relax.
8. Repeat 10 times.
9. Imagine tightening the muscles around your anus and pulling it up. Hold for a count of 5.
10. Relax.
11. Repeat 10 times.

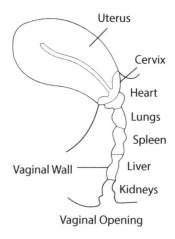

Figure 5.4. Zones of the Vagina

Exercise 5.4. Vertical Isolation

Next you can practice isolating the muscles up the vaginal canal.

1. Imagine that the entire canal, from entrance to cervix, is divided into five rings.
2. Practice tensing and releasing each ring up. Begin with the first ring; tense and release. Then the second ring; tense and release. The third ring; tense and release. The fourth ring; tense and release. And the fifth ring; tense and release.
3. Now work your way back down in the same fashion.
4. Repeat for 10 repetitions.

Exercise 5.5. Perineum Breathing [1]

In addition to strengthening the pelvic floor, perineum breathing can be used as a daily longevity exercise or for problems in the genital region for both men and women: yeast infections, low libido, UTI, menstrual issues, and prostate inflammation. Do not perform this exercise right before or after sex.

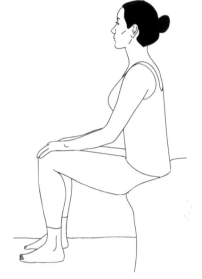

Figure 5.5. Perineum Breathing

1. Sit on the edge of a chair. Focus your attention on your perineum [2] and keep it there for the whole exercise.
2. Inhale. Pull the perineum up into the body (imagine a center line from your perineum to the top of your head). Hold for 2 seconds.
3. Exhale and relax completely.
4. Repeat for a total of 24 breaths.

Use of the Jade Egg

Pelvic floor exercises are highly effective, if performed correctly. Many women fail to achieve results because they are unable to adequately engage their muscles. Jade eggs were a tool used by ancient Daoists to facilitate mastery of the vaginal muscles. Using a jade egg provides instant feedback and resistance, just as lifting weights does versus performing bodyweight exercises. It also serves to increase sensitivity and body awareness within the vagina. Jade was chosen for its ability to nourish Yin. Modern women can choose jade eggs, eggs made of other types of stone, or ball-shaped vaginal weights. Any of these can be used for the exercises below. There are also biofeedback machines (as used in the French perineal re-education program) and electro-stimulators made for home use.

---

1. Modified from Merle Morgan-Drennan. "Medical Qigong" (lecture, Yo San University, Los Angeles, October 31, 2001). (student of Master Hong Liu)

2. Located between the genitals and anus.

Note: women need to exercise caution when inserting a jade egg or other strengthening tool in the vagina after delivery. You must first allow the skin in the genital region to fully heal from tears or sutures. When in doubt, ask your doctor.

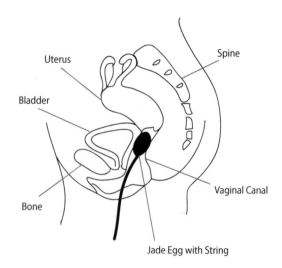

Figure 5.6. Inserting the Jade Egg

Choosing Your Egg

Choose your egg carefully. It should be made of a non-porous material such as a hard stone that can be sterilized. It should have a hole drilled through it. Dental floss or a sterile string is threaded through the hole and tied, with the tied end hanging outside of the vaginal, allowing for safe removal (like removing a tampon). As practice progresses, the string can be used to hang weights. Eggs come in three different sizes: small, medium, and large. Most women begin with a medium size and progress to a small one, which is more difficult to control. Women who have experienced vaginal delivery or muscle atrophy may prefer to begin with a large egg. The egg (or vaginal strengthening tool) should be small enough that it will slip out if the muscles are not activated, but large enough that holding it in is not too strenuous.

Always thoroughly disinfect a new stone egg by boiling it in vinegar and water for 15 minutes. Remove from the pot and cool prior to using. After every use, wash with mild soap and water and store in a clean dry place.

Exercise 5.6. Using a Jade Egg

This refines muscle control and sensitivity within the vagina. Repeat four to seven times a week.

1. Tie a piece of dental floss through the hole drilled in the egg. Make sure the tied end remains outside of your vagina. This allows you to safely remove it.
2. The egg is inserted wide-side first. Place at the opening of the vagina. Imagine the vaginal muscles pulling the egg inside the vagina as you gently push it in.
3. Practice tightening and relaxing your vaginal muscles and note how it feels different with the egg. As you contract your vaginal muscles imagine a central line connecting up to your heart and to the top of your head.
4. Next imagine moving the egg up the vaginal canal then back down again.
5. Repeat 10 times.
6. Imagine moving the egg horizontally from side to side.
7. To remove, imagine moving the egg out of the vagina while gently tugging on the string.

BENEFITS OF ADDING JADE EGGS

M. was a beautiful 35 year old mother of a two year old. She had been dribbling urine when she sneezed, laughed too hard, or picked up something heavy. M. thought it was normal right after delivery but the problem persisted. She had tried doing kegels but did not notice any difference in her symptoms. I treated her for Spleen and Kidney deficiency with acupuncture and herbs. I also recommended she try using a jade egg with weights four times a week. Within four weeks her symptoms were gone. M. also expressed a renewed interest in sex (she had not felt comfortable discussing before how she had lost any desire for sex).

I have had several such patients who came to me who had tried kegels and did not see results from them. When they took my suggestion to use a jade egg or other external weight they saw significant results within weeks.

Exercise 5.7. Jade Egg Weightlifting

This strongly strengthens the pelvic floor muscles. Repeat four times a week.

1. Place the jade egg in your vagina as before. Attach a weight to end of the floss and hold the floss so that your body does not feel the weight. (You can fill your jade egg bag with the remaining eggs or other stones).
2. Tighten your vaginal muscles and pull them up, as you slowly release the floss. Hold for a count of 5.
3. Hold the floss again relieving the weight from your vagina. Relax for a count of 10.
4. Again, tighten your vaginal muscles as you slowly release the floss. Hold for a count of 5.
5. Hold the floss again relieving the weight from your vagina. Relax for a count of 10.
6. Repeat until your muscles begin to fatigue. If you feel any discomfort, stop immediately and consult your doctor.

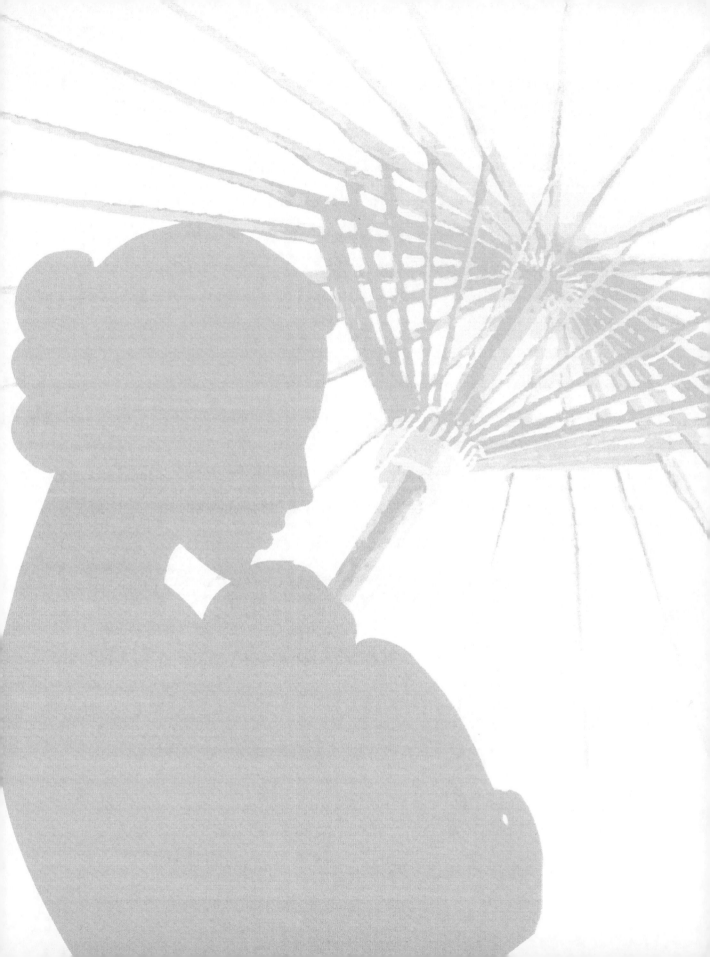

Chapter 6
Recovering the Abdomen

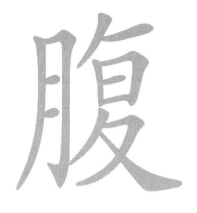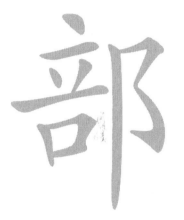

The muscles and connective tissue that comprise our core are the seat of our physical strength. They protect the vertebrae in our backs, allow us to safely lift objects, and maintain our posture. The abdomen is extremely vulnerable after childbirth. The expulsion of the fetus and placenta create a vacuum in the abdominal cavity. The abdominal muscles and connective tissue require rest and encouragement to go back to their pre-pregnancy state. Meanwhile, postpartum women are at risk of organ prolapse, which, compounded with pelvic floor weakness, can cause incontinence and other issues. Many of the practices in this chapter have been used for hundreds of years to protect women's internal organs from prolapse and displacement and to encourage full recovery of muscles and connective tissue.

These practices also have esthetic benefits. Without help, many women are left with loose skin, stretch marks, and damaged connective tissue. This damage is difficult to remedy after the postpartum months. Following these practices helps to fix the damage during a window of time when the body is readjusting.

Binding the Abdomen

After giving birth, the abdomen and internal organs need help returning to their original places. Abdominal binding performs two functions. First, it facilitates thorough healing of the abdomen: it minimizes the chances of organ prolapse, encourages the organs to go back to their rightful place, and supports healing of diastasis recti and C-section incisions (more on page 88). Second, it helps the mother recover esthetically, and improve her waistline. Without binding, new mothers can be left with a permanent puffy pooch.

When to Start
In cases of natural childbirth, begin the second day after giving birth. In case of C-section begin after the sixth day.

> ### A BALANCE BETWEEN MOBILITY & SUPPORT
> I once had a postpartum patient come in for treatment after throwing her back out from excessively tightening her girdle. It is best to slowly shrink the waist over 1-3 months.

When to Use and Duration
For the first 2 weeks, wear your girdle (or binding) 24 hours a day, removing it to bathe and eat. During the third, fourth, and fifth weeks, you can remove the girdle (or binding) at night. Wear it for at least one month after giving birth. For optimal esthetic results wear your girdle (or binding) for 3 months.

Postpartum Girdle vs. Abdominal Binding
There are pros and cons to manual binding and girdles. Girdles are convenient but less effective and binding is more effective but more labor intensive. Manually binding the abdomen allows for complete customization to a woman's body as it changes throughout the month. It is also inexpensive. However, it is harder and more time consuming to apply. Some women will not be able to do it themselves and will require assistance. This means someone who knows how to do abdominal binding will need to be there to reapply the binding at least once a day.

Many women prefer to buy a postpartum girdle. They are easy to put on and take off. Numerous options can be found on the internet at a range of costs. However, girdles do not offer the same customization. If you choose to use a girdle, look for one you can tighten and that covers your full abdomen, starting under the breasts to your pubic bone. The girdle should be firm without much give. Another option is to manually bind the abdomen for the first month or so, until the abdomen has regained much of its previous form, then switch to a postpartum girdle or full corset for the next two months.

Manual Binding

If you elect to do abdominal binding yourself, or have someone help you, you can cheat a little. For the first 2 weeks, remove the binding once a day to bathe, then reapply afterwards. Beginning the third week remove the binding at night, take a shower before bed or upon waking up, then reapply the binding in the morning.

1. **Binding Material** - Use a bandage or stretchy cloth that will allow the skin to breathe, about 10.4 yards in length and 5.5 inches in width. Women typically need three rolls of binding material at first and then go down to two. You may need more or less depending on your size and comfort. You can purchase traditional Taiwanese binding cloth at www. PostpartumRecoveryProgram.com.

2. **How Tight?** – You want to find a happy medium between support and mobility. The binding should feel snug. Your waist should feel smaller, your insides lifted, and your back supported. At the same time, you should not feel stifled, restricted, or irritated. You need to wear this binding for 24 hours so do not overdo it.

3. **Over Clothes?** – Here you have choice. If you apply the binding directly to your skin it will be less hot, but you will need to wash your binding. If you wear a thin undershirt or camisole, you can apply moisturizer to your abdomen or perspire without having to wash your binding. However, you will feel warmer and the binding can crimp the fabric of the undershirt making it uncomfortable.

4. **Binding Care** – Wash the binding material with cold water and line dry as needed to keep it clean. Keep the binding material rolled up after removing to preserve the shape for later use.

Exercise 6.1. Manual Abdominal Binding Instructions

1. Lie face up on your bed (or other comfortable place). Knees bent with your feet on the bed.

2. Lift up your hips into a mini bridge. Tuck your pelvis under slightly and maintain a slight contraction of your knees towards each other. This contraction will protect your back and promote contraction of your pelvic floor. If you feel too weak to hold this position, place 2 pillows under your hips and relax. This tilt is important to encourage lifting of the internal organs.

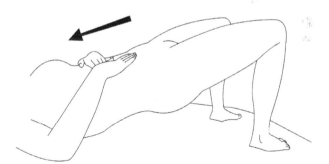

Figure 6.1. Massage the organs upwards toward the ribcage prior to manual binding or fastening the girdle.

3. Next, massage your abdominal organs up. To do this, press down on your lower abdomen with both hands, massaging upwards, bringing the internal organs toward the heart, stopping at the rib cage.

4. Begin wrapping from the pubic bone to the navel. (You will need 1-3 rolls for this).

5. Every round and a half make a slanting/oblique fold or twist with the bandage (Figure 6.3) in order to keep it from sliding, alternating side to side.

6. For the first 7 times around the lower torso, rise 1 inch with each round. After this, shift up 1 ½ inches with each round, spiraling up, with a final round past the navel then use a safety pin to fix the binding in place.

7. Now wrap the upper abdomen. (You will need 1-2 rolls for this). Begin the first round overlapping the last round of the lower bandage.

   a. Use the same technique as with the lower abdomen. Make a twist with the bandage every 1 ½ rounds, alternating side to side.

   b. Shift up 1 ½ inches after each round.

Note: If you are very thin and your hipbones protrude, add padding to the lower abdomen, like a towel, before binding. The binding material should be kept rolled up after removing to preserve the shape for later use.

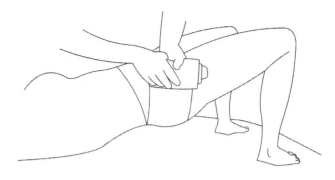

Figure 6.2. Begin wrapping just above the pubic bone and work up to underneath the breasts.

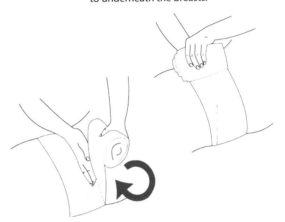

Figure 6.3. Make an oblique fold or twist every 1 1/2 rounds. In other words, alternate which side of the torso you make the fold.

Postpartum Girdle

A postpartum girdle offers convenience. Be sure to adhere to the following tips:

1. **Choosing a Girdle** - There are two main criteria for choosing a girdle. First, it should be adjustable to accommodate your changing body. Second, it must cover your full abdomen, from your pubic bone all the way to below your breasts. Taiwanese and Chinese postpartum girdles often come in three pieces to accommodate different bodies. These can be purchased on www.PostpartumRecoveryProgram.com, however the sizes are too small for many Western women.

2. **How Tight?** – You want to find a happy medium between support and mobility. The binding should feel snug. Your waist should feel smaller, your insides lifted, and your back supported. At the same time, you should not feel stifled, restricted, or irritated. You need to wear this binding for 24 hours so do not overdo it.

3. **Over Clothes?** – It is more convenient to wear your girdle over a thin undershirt or camisole, unless you purchase more than one girdle and wash them often.
4. **Girdle Care** – Wash the girdle by hand with cold water and dry it flat as needed to keep it clean.

Exercise 6.2. Applying a Postpartum Girdle

When using a postpartum girdle follow the same guidelines for abdominal binding. Be sure to continue to keep the abdomen moisturized to minimize stretch marks.

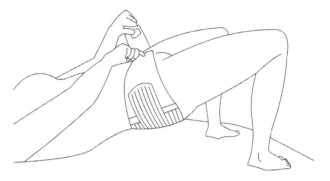

Figure 6.4. Begin wrapping the lower abdomen.

1. Lie face up on your bed (or other comfortable place). Knees bent with your feet on the bed.
2. Lift up your hips into a mini bridge. Tuck your pelvis under slightly and maintain a slight contraction of your knees towards each other. This contraction will protect your back and promote contraction of your pelvic floor. If you feel too weak to hold this position, place 2 pillows under your hips and relax. This tilt is important to encourage lifting of the internal organs.

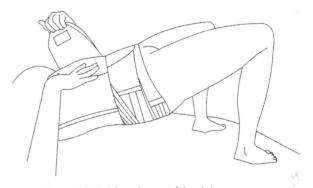

Figure 6.5. Finish at the top of the abdomen.

3. Next, massage your abdominal organs up. To do this, press down on your lower abdomen with both hands, massaging upwards, bringing the internal organs toward the heart, stopping at the rib cage.
4. Begin binding the girdle, beginning at the pubic bone and finishing at the ribcage.

You want to apply the girdle firmly, but not too tightly. Be sure you can breathe and move around (somewhat) comfortably. **Note:** Continue to apply rich oils to the abdomen daily for the first 2 months postpartum to avoid stretch marks.

Protecting the Abdomen

Restrict Activity

The restrictions on lifting will seem archaic and excessive, but they are necessary to protect the pelvic floor, abdomen (especially after a C-section), and joints. In addition to the vulnerability of the abdomen and pelvic floor discussed above, women's ligaments are lax postpartum due to the changes in hormones. This weakens the joints, particularly in the low back and knees.

Do Not Climb Stairs

Avoid going up and down stairs for the entire 30-40 days. This is especially important for women who have a C-section. Going up and down stairs can cause stiches in the abdomen to open. Additionally, the low back and joints are vulnerable after birth.

Do Not Lift Weight

This means avoiding weightlifting and picking up anything heavy. There are two reasons. First, you need to conserve your energy. Second, straining can cause organ prolapse. The intra-abdominal pressure when you engage your core sends pressure down on the pelvic floor. Have your helpers do any lifting for you as much as possible. Avoid weight training for 30-40 days. Return to weight training very slowly and cautiously for six months after giving birth. (See exercises page 88).

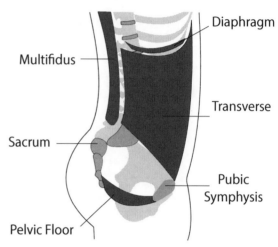

Figure 6.6. Core Muscles

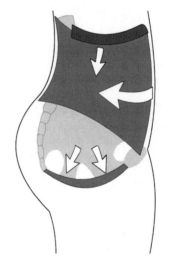

Figure 6.7. Intra-abdominal Pressure

Athletes and Avid Exercisers

If you were used to high intensity exercises before, you will be eager to get back to them. Begin with muscle control, calisthenics-type exercises, and walking. If you have this personality, focus on getting crazy strong pelvic floor muscles. After the first month, slowly begin to resume your exercises at regular intensity. Focus on maintaining function, strength, stimulating blood flow, and emotional well-being. Do not establish any new fitness goals beyond recovering your previous form for the first six months postpartum.

Avoid cardio exercises entirely the first month. Excessive strain and sweating can easily create Qi and Yin deficiency. Slowly resume cardio after the 30-40 days. Wait four to six months to resume intense cardio training.

Most Important to Avoid During the Postpartum Recovery Program™:
1. Exercises that cause a high degree of intra-abdominal pressure, such as lifting heavy weights, pullups, pushups, and planks.
2. Deep squats.
3. Strenuous abdominal workouts. Bending the abdominals.
4. Cardio.

General Exercise

If you want an at-home DVD for your postpartum month use one specific for postpartum women or for women with prolapse. I recommend the following:

1. Callanetics series of videos except for the cardio. These utilize muscle control exercises with a focus on the pelvic floor.[1]
2. Michelle Canway's exercise DVD. She is a physiotherapist who focuses on pelvic floor rehabilitation.[2]
3. There are yoga and Pilates instructors who focus on pelvic floor rehabilitation. There are videos available such as Your Pace Yoga DVD.

Do Not Carry Your Baby

For the same reasons you should not lift weights. Have someone else carry and bathe your baby, preferably your partner or other family member to encourage bonding.

Lie on Your Side to Nurse

Lie on your side propped with pillows so that you are very comfortable. Have someone carry the baby to you.

---

1. Available at www.callanetics.com
2. Available at www.pelvicexercises.com.au

Strengthening the Abdominal Muscles

Once you have learned how to engage the pelvic floor you can begin engaging your abdominals. How quickly you can progress with abdominal strengthening depends on the condition of your abdomen.

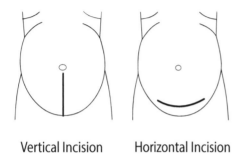

Vertical Incision   Horizontal Incision

Figure 6.8. A transverse incision is preferred for speed of healing and cosmetic results. A vertical incision is sometimes necessary as it provides speedier access during an emergency and allows for a greater opening.

Are You Recovering From a C-Section?

If you had a C-section you must wait until your doctor has checked your incisions and clears you for abdominal exercises (typically 6-8 weeks). After you have been cleared, begin exercises slowly at low intensity, and build up from there as long as there is no discomfort. Stay tuned in to your body at all times. Exercising too early can cause the sutures to spilt open leaving long-term ramifications.

Do You Have Diastasis Recti?

Diastasis recti is a separation on the midline of the rectus abdominis muscle. The expansion of the abdomen during pregnancy can overstretch the connective tissue (linea alba) between the right and left rectus abdominis muscles, causing it to tear.

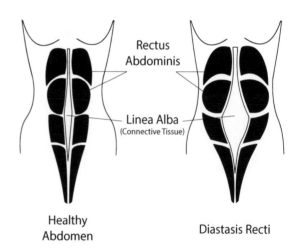

Rectus Abdominis

Linea Alba (Connective Tissue)

Healthy Abdomen

Diastasis Recti

Figure 6.9. Normal abdomen and abdomen with diastasis recti.

Exercise 6.3. Self-Test for Diastasis Recti:

4. Lie on your back with your knees bent. Place the fingers of your left hand above belly button and the fingers of your right hand below you belly button.
5. Raise your head and shoulders off floor.
6. Feel the centerline of your abdomen. Is there a vertical separation between the right and left rectus abdominis muscle? If there is you will feel a gap in the muscle right along the

centerline or a bulge. If there is a separation, take note of the following:

a. What is the location of the separation? Is it above or below the belly button?

b. To assess the degree of the rupture, turn your four fingers towards your feet and place in the area of the separation (Figure 6.9). How many fingers can you place in the gap, one – two – three – four? Placing one to two fingers in the gap is normal. If you can place more than two fingers in the gap, you have diastasis recti.

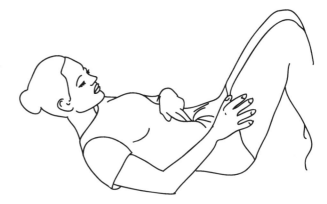

Figure 6.10. Diastasis recti self-test.

If you feel an indentation, then you should wait until the muscle heals prior to doing abdominal exercises. Continue wearing your postpartum girdle and eat collagen-rich bone broth soups to speed the process. In severe cases surgery is required to re-attach the muscle. Consult your doctor for advice.

Exercise 6.4. Connecting with Your Core

The purpose of this exercise is to get your core to work synergistically and safely.

1. Lie face up with your knees bent and your feet on the floor.
2. Press your heels into the ground to activate your buttocks, but do not lift up your hips. Press your knees towards each other to activate the inner thighs and pelvic floor. Lift the entire pelvic floor up towards your head.
3. Once you have your entire pelvic floor engaged and lifted, press the backs of your arms into the ground, and slide your scapula down your back to engage your latisimus dorsi.
4. Finally, bring your lower ribs towards each other and down towards your pubic bone.
5. Relax completely.

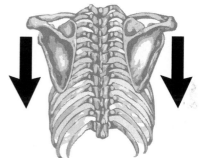

Figure 6.11. Engage the scapulas.

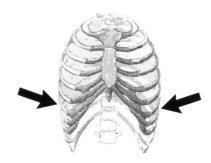

Figure 6.12. Engage the ribcage.

6. This time do not tense your legs or buttocks. Tighten your pelvic floor and lift it up towards your head as high as you can.
7. Press the backs of your arms into the ground, and slide your scapula down your back to engage your latisimus dorsi.
8. Finally, bring your lower ribs towards each other and down towards your pubic bone.
9. Relax completely.
10. Repeat for a total of 10-20 repetitions. Once you can complete 20 repetitions comfortably, progress to the Quarter Crunch and Transverse Abdominis Raise below.

If there is any discomfort stop and wait to attempt abdominal exercises.

Exercise 6.5. Quarter Crunch

The quarter crunch is a safe abdominal exercise that predominantly engages the rectus abdominis.

1. Lie face up with your knees bent and your feet on the floor. Arms at your sides.
2. Tighten your pelvic floor and lift it up towards your head as high as you can.
3. Slide your scapula down your back to engage your latisimus dorsi.
4. Bring your lower ribs towards each other and down towards your pubic bone (When you master this contraction, you will feel your solar plexus, the abdominal space between your ribs, engage and get tight). Allow the abdominal contraction to bring your head, shoulders, and arms off the floor.
5. Relax completely.
6. Repeat for a total of 10-20 repetitions.

Exercise 6.6. Transverse Abdominis Raise [3]

This exercise strengthens the transverse abdominis; the deep abdominal muscles that play a key part in core strength.

1. Get on your hands and knees. Align your shoulders over your hands and your hips over your knees.
2. Keep your head straight and spine in neutral position.
3. Breathe out.
4. Tighten the pelvic floor and draw it up.

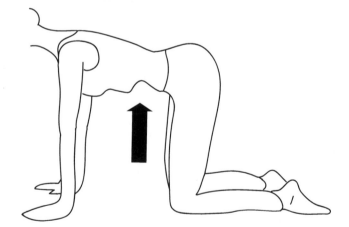

Figure 6.13. Transverse Abdominal Raise.

3. Retrieved from www.bacinfo.com/2010/04/01/bac-training-tip-transverse-abdominus-raise

5. Draw your belly button in towards the spine (do not round your back). Hold for a count of 5. Do not hold your breath, but breathe in and out normally.
6. Relax, breathing normally.
7. Repeat for 20 repetitions.

I recommend getting a series of private classes from an experienced Pilates instructor or other training coach with experience in training postpartum women. Women trainers who have gone through the process of reconnecting with their core muscles after a C-section are a good choice.

Recovering Your Waist

In addition to wearing a postpartum girdle and reconnecting with your abdominal muscles, some women find an abdominal massage helpful. A massage therapist trained in postpartum abdominal massage can relax tight muscles and support the movement of organs back to their rightful place.

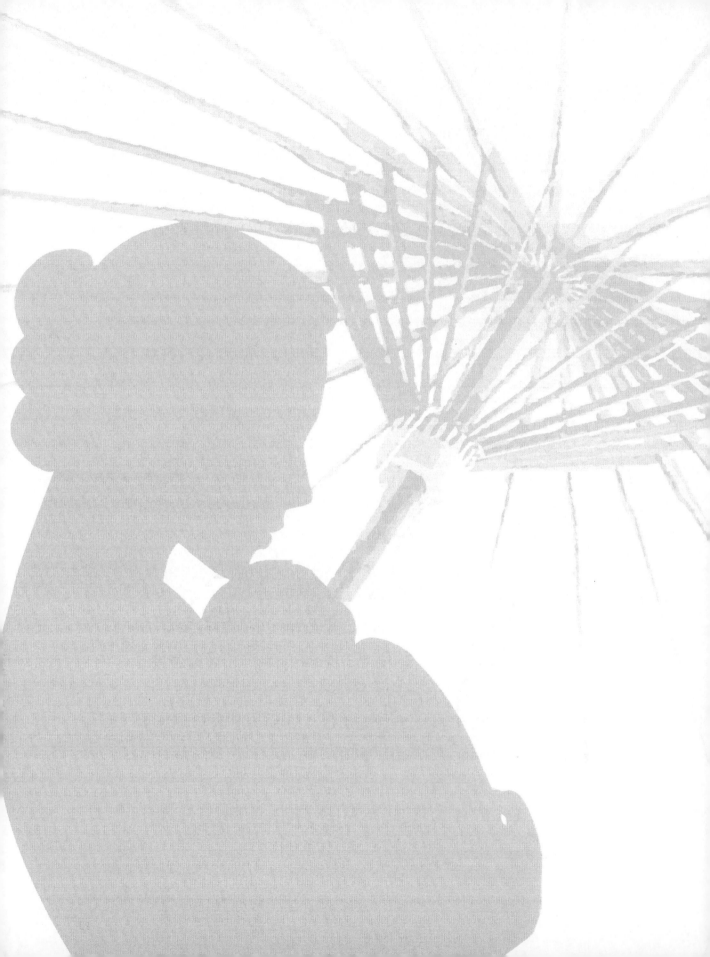

Chapter 7
Breast Care

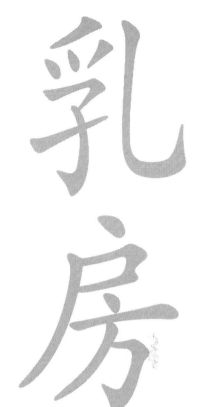

Breast Feeding

Ideally mothers should breastfeed for four months. Some recommend one year during which time the baby should not have any meat[1] while others recommend beginning weaning any time after the first four months.[2] Many women benefit from consulting a lactation coach (a role which may be filled by a midwife or doula). Do not rely on hospital staff to provide this service.

Following the Postpartum Recovery Plan™ will strengthen the mother and promote healthy milk production. From the first two weeks postpartum until you stop breastfeeding, eat milk-promoting recipes at least three times a week. These include ingredients such as carp, green papaya, peanuts, and pork trotters that build Qi and Blood in the body.[3] If there is low milk production in spite of

---

1. Jiang Zheng. "TCM Gynecology." (lecture, Pacific College of Oriental Medicine, San Diego, January 20, 2007).
2. From author's synopsis of an interview by Veronica Anover with Dr. Stéphane Marmié, August 2013.
3. Jiang Zheng. "TCM Gynecology." (lecture, Pacific College of Oriental Medicine, San Diego, January 20, 2007).

this, seek help from an acupuncturist. When you wish to stop lactating, use Roasted Sprouted Barley Tea (page 161). Drink one cup, three times a day for three days.

It is common for new mothers to feel guilty if their plans of breastfeeding "fail." There are situations beyond a mother's control which can impede breastfeeding such as having a tongue-tied infant (ankyloglossia), a condition where the frenulum is too short or extends excessively restricting movement of the tongue. In some cases an experienced lactation coach or physician can remedy the situation, and other times they cannot. Breast feeding is only one factor in securing the health of your baby.

A CASE OF "IT IS NEVER TOO LATE"

J. was overwhelmed by a difficult birth experience, compounded by breastfeeding issues and a philandering husband. Six months later her menses returned heavy and irregular. J. returned to get treatments very sporadically, limited by the demands of single motherhood. Four years after the birth of her baby, J. walked into my clinic looking a strong woman, if a bit frazzled, stressed, and overworked.

She began practicing Inner Alchemy breast massage,[1] getting regular acupuncture, and started wearing a postpartum girdle. She also started Pilates classes. She took a patent formula (due to convenience) called Return to Spring.[2] Her period was at first more irregular, then settled into a regular cycle after three months. Her menstrual flow was comfortably lighter and shortened to four days.

---

1. Lia Andrews. *7 Times a Woman; Ancient Wisdom on Health & Beauty Every Woman Should Know.* (San Diego: Alcyone Press, 2013), 139.

2. *Huan Shao Dan* is a Kidney tonic that also strengthens the Spleen and calms the Shen.

Breast Health

Cracked Nipple

Nipples can get bruised up from breast feeding. It is common to experience bruising, cuts, and even bleeding.

1. **Apply moisturizing salves** to the nipples after breast feeding to prevent chaffing.
2. **Use Zi Cao Oil or Balm.** Zi Cao (Radix Arnebiae seu Lithospermi) speeds healing, calms inflammation, and is anti-bacterial.

Thrush on the Nipple

Thrush occurs when there is *Candida albicans* (yeast) overgrowth in mouth. This overgrowth happens when the immune system is depressed, when antibiotics kill off healthy flora that keep

Candida in check, and/or there is excessive moisture or consistent micro-trauma to an area. It is a common occurrence in infants and can be passed on to the mother's nipple. To treat it, you can:

1. **Make a Yin Care compress.** As mentioned above, Yin Care is a concentrated decoction of anti-fungal Chinese Herbs. Dilute with water in a bowl and saturate in sterile gauze or 2x4 cotton rounds. Place over the nipple for 10 minutes daily for 7 consecutive days.
2. **Apply Huang Lian Gao (Coptis Ointment) or Huang Lian (coptis) powder after breastfeeding.** This is a less time consuming option. Huang Lian (coptis) is a broad spectrum anti-fungal, anti-bacterial, and anti-viral herb.

Mastitis

Mastitis is an infection of the breast tissue and is a common postpartum malady.

To prevent mastitis:

1. Beginning during pregnancy, Gu Sha (Figure 7.1) both breasts daily from the outside in towards the nipples. Either apply oil or place a piece of silk over the skin to avoid tugging the skin. Apply firm pressure and use a scraping movement until the skin pinks up.
2. After childbirth, immediately begin massaging any nodules in the breast to soften them. This may be painful at first. Once the baby begins to nurse, nodules will be dispersed. Continue daily Gua Sha and massage for the duration of breast feeding.
3. At the first signs of inflammation or pain, seek help from an acupuncturist. You can also make a strong decoction (60g) of coix seeds (*yi yi ren*) and drink liberally.
4. If the problem does not resolve quickly, seek medical attention. If it develops into a full-blown infection you may require antibiotics.

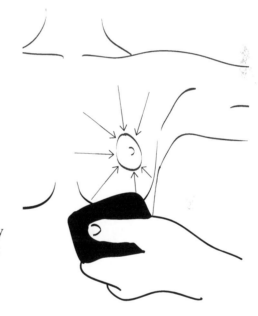

Figure 7.1. Gua Sha for Mastitis

Recovering Breast Tissue

It is common to hear that women will lose a breast size with every child and the breasts will sag after breastfeeding. In Traditional Chinese Medicine, sagging breasts are the result of Qi and Blood deficiency. Following postpartum recovery, limiting the length of breast feeding, and not becoming depleted will prevent cosmetic changes to the breasts. If sagging or loss of tissue has already occurred, get a customized herbal formula from an acupuncturist and do the breast massage techniques below:

Exercise 7.1. Breast Massage Protocol

Perform exercises daily. If performed correctly the skin will pink up. This indicates sufficient blood flow to the skin. Be sure to apply oil to the breasts prior to performing the exercises.

Knuckling
Make loose fists. Use your knuckles to massage working up the lines shown in Figure 7.2. Work deeply until the skin pinks up. It will be borderline painful at first as there will be more stagnation (like deep tissue massage.) To affect the deeper tissues that you want to get to, you have to be a bit aggressive.

Pinching
Next use your thumb and index finger to pinch up the lines shown in Figure 7.3. Again work deeply, really grabbing the tissue. Always work up.

Slapping
Slap the breast tissue working up.

Hot and Cold
Hot and cold therapy will greatly increase circulation and flush out waste material from the cells. Alternate ice water compresses with warm water compresses.

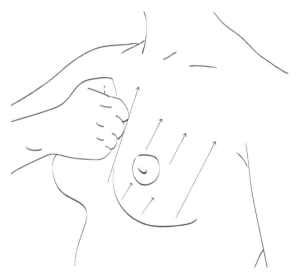

Figure 7.2. Knuckling

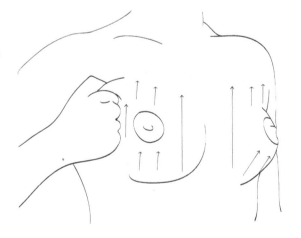

Figure 7.3. Pinching

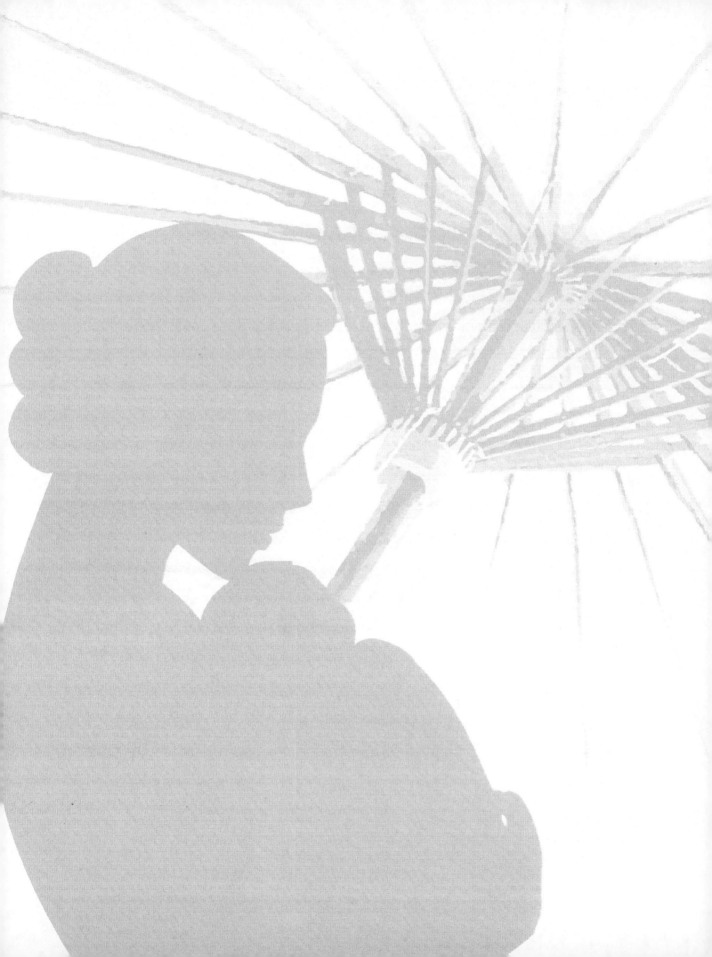

Chapter 8

Healing Birth Trauma

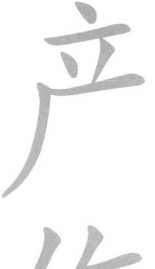

Healing requires energy. Thus, a main focus of postpartum recovery is to strengthen the body to recover quickly and prevent infection. There are instances where the body suffers additional damage during childbirth and requires more help to heal itself. In this chapter we cover common postpartum injuries along with remedies you can use at home. If your body is not recovering as expected you should consult your physician and acupuncturist.

Vaginal Care

Lochia

For 2-4 weeks after birth, women pass lochia, a mixture of blood, mucous, and uterine tissue. To many, it is like a medium to heavy period. Chinese herbs and acupuncture treatments are given to pass the lochia quickly and completely. Residual stagnation of lochia can lead to long-term gynecological issues. Abdominal pain can be a sign of lochial retention. Additionally, lochia lasting more than 4-6 weeks can be a sign of infection.

Vaginal Trauma

The genital region will be sore and puffy after a vaginal delivery. The vagina will have been stretched to capacity, causing micro-tears in the musculature and skin that must be repaired. Vaginal tears occur in anywhere from 40-79% of vaginal births. Additionally, some women elect to have or require an episiotomy.

Degrees:
1. **First Degree Tear** – is a superficial tear that occurs around the perineum and opening of the vagina. It involves only the skin and not the muscles. It requires few or no stitches and heals quickly.
2. **Second Degree Tear** – is a deeper tear that affects the muscle layer and must be stitched layer by layer. It causes more discomfort and takes weeks to heal.
3. **Third Degree Tear** – is a tear that extends to the anus.
4. **Fourth Degree Tear** – is a tear that goes through the anal sphincter and the tissue underneath it.
5. **Obstetric Fistula** – If labor becomes obstructed (i.e. a newborn is stuck in the birth canal) and labor extends beyond three days it can cause lack of blood flow to parts of the vaginal wall. This leads to necrosis (cell death) and creates holes extending from the birth canal into the intestinal wall and/or the bladder leading to fecal and or urinary incontinence. This is a major health issue for women in areas without adequate medical care and can be avoided by performing a timely C-section.[1]

There are several natural remedies you can use to speed healing and ease discomfort:
1. **Colloidal Silver** – can be diluted with water and used as a compress to ease swelling, disinfect wounds, and speed healing. To make a compress mix colloidal silver with water in a bowl. Soak sterile gauze or cotton 2x4s in liquid and place on the genital area for 10 minutes. If the vaginal area feels hot to the touch (is inflamed) you can use ice water with colloidal silver. Colloidal silver can also be used as a spray. The colloidal silver compress can also be used for skin issues your baby may have including rashes and eczema.
2. **Yunnan Baiyao**[2] – is a well-known TCM first aid remedy for numerous ailments. Yunnan Baiyao moves the Blood, stops excess bleeding, eases pain, and disinfects. It comes in several forms: pills for internal use, powder for external use, spray for injuries, and plasters for muscle soreness. The powder can be sprinkled onto tears and cuts to prevent infection, stop bleeding, reduce swelling, and speed healing. Take capsules internally, daily to prevent scar tissue formation. Take as directed by your acupuncturist. Contraindicated with certain medications such as blood thinners.
3. **Zi Cao Oil or Balm** – is another well-known remedy for burns, tears, bruises, or any inflammatory skin condition, including diaper rash. It contains Zi Cao (Radix Arnebiae

---

1. For more on this topic visit www.fistulafoundation.org/what-is-fistula or watch a documentary on the subject at www.pbs.org/wgbh/nova/body/a-walk-to-beautiful.html

2. Be sure to purchase Yunnan Baiyao with blue or green labeling. Camelia brand Yunnan Baiyao with the yellow and pink labeling has degraded significantly in quality and efficacy in the last few years.

seu Lithospermi) as the main ingredient, which imparts its characteristic red-purple color, and can include other herbs. Zi Cao Oil clears Heat (inflammation or burning pain), clears Heat Toxin (infection), and Damp-Heat (itchy or fluid-filled rashes). Apply Zi Cao Oil to the genital area to reduce swelling and speed healing. For increased strength you can mix Zi Cao Oil with Yunnan Baiyao powder and apply.

4. **Huang Lian Gao** – is anti-bacterial and anti-fungal. It can be used like Zi Cao Oil above. Additionally it is used to treat thrush on the nipples.

5. **Yin Care** – Hormonal imbalances and antibiotic use can trigger yeast infections.[3] Yin Care is a concentrated decoction of anti-fungal herbs that is used as a douche or poultice to quickly alleviate yeast infection symptoms. If you have had a vaginal delivery, you should not use a douche for 6 weeks or so. If there is no trauma to the vaginal wall, a tampon can be soaked in the solution and inserted into the vagina for 1 hour daily for 7 consecutive days. Your TCM herbalist can also give you a tea you can brew and sit over, allowing the herbal steam to penetrate the tissue. This is called a sitz bath and is the ideal method to treat the condition, though it is more labor intensive and time consuming. Vaginal suppositories made of Chinese herbs are also available from many acupuncturists.

C-Section Healing

C-sections save the genitals from trauma, but they constitute major surgery and introduce other issues. Namely scar tissue formation and adhesions. These can cause loss of sensation, mobility, loss of muscle connection, or pain. It is especially important to wear a postpartum girdle for at least 5-6 weeks if you had a C-section. You must avoid stairs, lifting anything over 20 lbs. and abdominal exercises for 6 weeks or until you are cleared by your physician. This is to avoid breaking the stitches which creates further complications. Additionally, you will want to take herbs to prevent the formation of scar tissue and minimize visible scarring.

Minimizing Internal Scar Tissue Formation

1. **Yunnan Baiyao Capsules** [4] – take daily after C-section to prevent scar tissue formation. Take as directed by your acupuncturist. Contraindicated with certain medications such as blood thinners.

2. **Avogen Capsules** – an avocado extract that breaks up scar tissue. Take 1 capsule (40mg), once per day beginning in the second trimester of pregnancy and continuing on until 3 months postpartum.[5]

---

3. Yeast infections occur when the immune system is suppressed and Candida albicans, a microorganism present in our bodies, proliferates beyond normal numbers. If this occurs in the mouth it is called thrush. If it occurs in the vagina it is called a yeast infection. If it occurs throughout the body it is called systemic candidiasis. Typical yeast infection symptoms are vaginal itching and a cottage cheese-like white discharge.

4. Avoid Camellia Brand (in the yellow and pink box) which has gone down in quality. Instead use Yunnan Baiyao in a green and white or blue and white box.

5. Dr. Richard Huber, founder of Avogen USA and 302 Professional Skincare. Avogen is available at www.AvogenUSA.com.

3. **Acupuncture and Herbal Medicine** – can speed healing and minimize scar tissue formation.

4. **Endermologie™ Treatments** – are performed with a machine utilizing suction, a rolling action, and tapotement that drains the lymphatic system, increases microcirculation, and breaks up scar tissue and fatty deposits. Endermologie also treats postpartum edema and weight gain. It is very effective performed 1-2 times a week on healed scars.

Minimizing Visible Scarring

1. **Yunnan Baiyao Liquid**[6] – apply topically on scars. Take internally as well as directed by your acupuncturist. Contraindicated with certain medications such as blood thinners. Consult your acupuncturist prior to using.

2. **Avogen Mist**[7] – contains Avogen. Softens scar tissue, increases circulation, and rejuvenates the skin.

3. **Acupuncture and Microneedling** – breaks up scar tissue and rejuvenates the skin.

4. **Ultrasound Treatments** – performed weekly over several months can minimize stretch marks and scarring.

---

6. Avoid Camellia Brand (in the yellow and pink box) which has gone down in quality. Instead use Yunnan Baiyao in a green and white or blue and white box.

7. Alternately, 302 Drops can be used topically, but is only sold through licensed professionals.

Emotional Healing

Resuming Your Identity
In French culture, women are expected to get their identity back as women three months after having a baby; including being a sexual being. In American culture, however, being a mom is often perceived as an all-consuming, exclusive identity. The Postpartum Recovery Program™ will help you recover your strength and your body. You must also develop a new identity that includes you as a whole being and mother.

Postpartum Depression

Some women are on an oxytocin high for months after they have their baby. For others, the drop in hormones, Qi and Blood deficiency, Blood stasis, the physical changes to their body, along with the major lifestyle adjustment a new baby brings sends them into a depression. Women are often not aware they are slipping into depression, and many doctors do not spend enough time with patients to pick up on signs, so it is often up to family and friends to intervene. Though postpartum recovery does a great deal to prevent postpartum depression, it is not enough in some cases. In TCM there are two major reasons for postpartum depression, or baby blues; Blood deficiency and Blood stasis.

Blood Deficiency Postpartum Depression
Symptoms: fatigue, weakness, guilt, easy to cry, feeling unsupported and isolated.

Treatment: This type of depression responds well to customized herbal formulas given by acupuncturists and acupuncture treatment. Be sure to get 8-10 hours of sleep, eat lactation-promoting soups, and eat sufficient protein.

Blood Stasis Postpartum Depression
Symptoms: psychosis, lack of bonding with baby, suicidal thoughts, aggression, and irrational thinking.

Treatment: This type of depression is more severe and typically requires medical intervention. Medication is often needed in order to jumpstart recovery, after which herbal medicine, acupuncture, qigong, yoga, and other natural methods can be used.

Sisterhood

Recent years have seen the emergence of supportive communities, both in person and online, where women can vent, give advice, and problem solve. It has also created venues for unconsciousness to express its venom anonymously, and meanness and bullying abound on the internet. Many of us women are still working through our knee jerk reaction to judge other women harshly.[8] Do not take it personally if a sister tells you to suck it up or judges you. She likely never got the support she needed herself.

8. An excellent book on indirect aggression amongst women is Phyllis Chesler. *Woman's Inhumanity to Woman.* (Chicago: Lawrence Hill Books, 2009).

KAREN'S STORY: HOW ONE WOMAN CLIMBED HER WAY OUT

During her first pregnancy, Karen had nausea but it was manageable. She had continued working full-time up until a week before delivery and was back to work three months after having her baby. Her first son never latched on, so Karen pumped and bottle fed for six weeks. The nurse at the hospital had gotten frustrated with her and said, "I don't know how you'll ever do this." This made Karen more committed to breast feed her second child.

Karen's second pregnancy was a unique experience. Her depression crept in while she was still pregnant. She had been very sick from the beginning of her pregnancy. She could not get out of bed, felt constant nausea, had to get hydration IVs, and lost 10 lbs. during her first trimester. Karen did not respond to treatments. She got scared when she began her second trimester and the nausea was still there. Only after 20 weeks did the nausea finally subside on its own.

"I had already given up on doing the pregnancy the way I wanted: eating organic healthy food, having a natural birth, breastfeeding, etc. The reality was in my first trimester I was so nauseated I couldn't even take prenatal vitamins," Karen said. She remembered a two day period where she ate a box of donuts, which was all she could keep down. She felt like a failure, so she gave up on natural birth. She tried to be natural during her pregnancy, but had to be on medications. She had wanted to try acupuncture but it was not covered by insurance. By the time she delivered her baby she was already depleted. Karen did not feel compassion from the hospital staff and she just wanted to get home to recover. She did not have a midwife or doula.

After the birth Karen spiraled down. Her husband, who traveled frequently, took 10 days off from work to be with her. He tried to be supportive but he did not understand what was happening or how to help. Karen felt disappointed that no one, other than her mom and husband, had stepped in to help, especially the women in her life who were also mothers. Her mother was sympathetic, as she had also suffered from depression, but was physically unable to help as much as she wanted. Her mother-in-law had had three children under the age of 5 and could not understand why Karen "couldn't get it together."

Karen stayed home with her second child but rather than make things easier, her recovery was much harder. Karen developed anxiety about going places and breastfeeding in public. Breastfeeding was worse with her second son. She was producing so much milk but her son was tongue-tied. She continued trying for one month to no avail. This intensified her isolation. She felt she was being judged when she spoke with doctors and nurses on the issue. She became so sensitive to the question of breast feeding. She felt she had to explain she was not a bad mom. She also felt like a failure because she had not enjoyed her pregnancy. She had failed at her own expectation of herself. Other people did not understand why she was so upset over this. Her husband would tell her to "put it behind you." He did not make her feel guilty but he also could not relate to her feelings.

The depression came in waves. The first spell lasted from the birth of her second son in September to January. Karen began menstruating by the second month postpartum. She had extreme fatigue, bad insomnia, night sweats, and rushes of heat in her upper body. She could only sleep when her baby slept. She was prescribed Prozac (an anti-depressant) but did not respond well, so she was put on Zoloft instead along with the anti-anxiety medication Ativan. These made her feel like she was in a fog, but they helped her find some kind of normalcy. The depression seemed to subside.

Then in April her mood dipped again badly. Her husband decided to hire a nanny. Karen was against it because of money issues and was embarrassed she needed the help. She was a stay at home mom and felt she should be able to handle it. They hired a nanny in May, six months after delivery, to come in twice a week, when Karen's mom developed health issues and she had additional caregiving responsibilities.

She stayed on Zoloft for 1½ years and it took a full two years to recover. The medication kick-started her recovery and made her functional, but once she started seeing her way out she made the choice to seek help elsewhere. Yoga classes gave her something to look forward to. She met nice people. Making it to class became a goal and she enrolled in teacher training classes.

When I met Karen she was a glowing woman who decided to funnel her desire for a big family into fostering and adopting more children. She saw her experience as bestowing her with a great deal of compassion and wisdom. She certainly would not tell a woman in need to toughen up. It was also a blessing in that it opened her to adoption. Her experience had brought her a passion for teaching prenatal yoga, so that other moms can have a different experience. Her advice to expectant moms is to know ahead of time exactly what you want and verbalize it. Karen now owns a company she started with a friend who is a lactation consultant. They are teaming up to offer private and small group prenatal yoga and lactation education, as well as, Mom and Baby yoga classes for postnatal moms. Her main intention is to help mother's prepare their bodies and minds for childbirth and postpartum so that they hopefully will not have to go through what she went through.

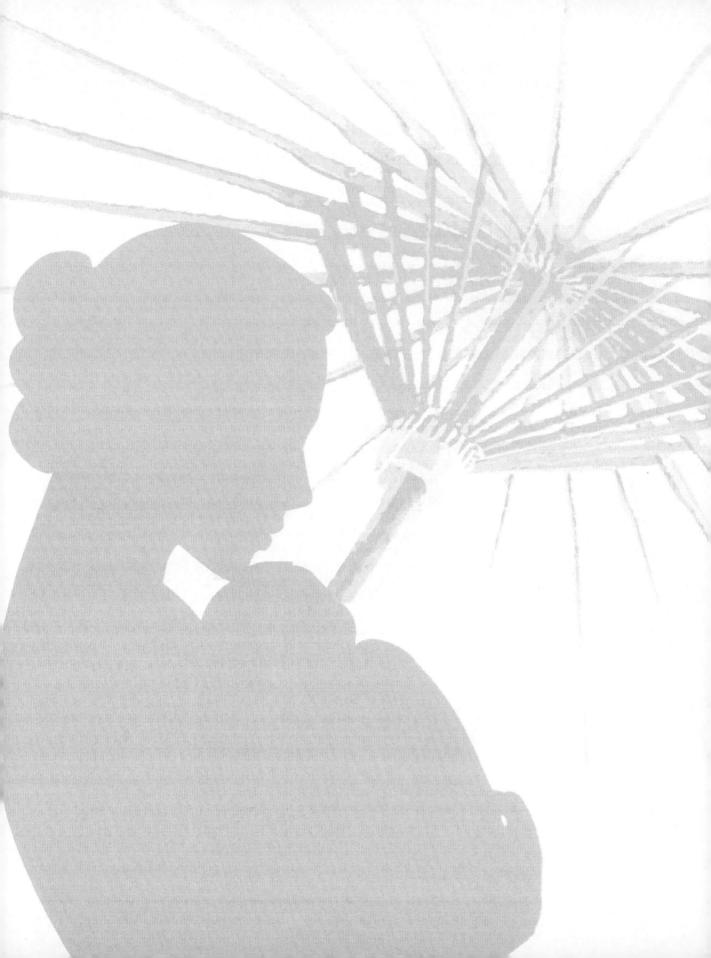

Chapter 9
Sexuality

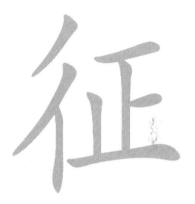

Sexuality and relationship are areas that require adjustment postpartum. Besides the physical changes, you may be out of sorts emotionally and in terms of energy.

Romantic Relationship

It is common for your partner to feel left out of the birth and postpartum process. He or she should take a central role in the Postpartum Recovery Program™ and be made to feel special as well. Your partner must also show up and support you. It is during these times that we discover who is really with us through life's turns.

Sex After a Baby

Sexual intercourse is restricted for six weeks postpartum. It is also necessary to recover your physical strength, particularly your Kidney Qi, prior to expending sexual energy. Besides the physical impediments, body image issues, fatigue, and new parental roles can undermine a healthy libido.

How you feel about yourself is the biggest indicator of how you will be received. Love yourself, love your body, delight in your sexuality, and expect your partner to receive you in kind.

1. Maintain loving connection, physical affection, and thoughtful acts with your partner. This connection is necessary for most women to have sexual desire.
2. Begin with non-intercourse sex. It is normal to fear penetration after vaginal delivery. First try other forms of sexual connection that feel safe and comfortable.
3. Resuming intercourse. Many women express feeling like they have a different body during sex. You might go through a period of rediscovering what works and what does not.
4. If there is pain there is a problem. If you experience pain after the second or third time of intercourse there may be an issue with scar tissue formation or poorly healing tears. You should seek help from your doctor.

How to Flow Sexual Energy & Strengthen the Low Back

One of my teachers, Dr. Mingdong Li, swore by this simple exercise to strengthen sexual vitality, tonify the Kidneys, and keep the low back and hips healthy and supple. This makes it an excellent exercise to do postpartum. Dr. Li advocated everyone perform 100 repetitions daily.[1]

Exercise 9.1. Pelvic Circles

1. Stand with your feet together. Bend your knees slightly. Bend at the hips and place your hands on your knees.
2. Begin performing hip circles. To start, stick you hip out to the right, then to the front, then to the left, then back. Once you get comfortable, try to smooth out the movement. Perform 50 circles.
3. Repeat going the other way 50 times.

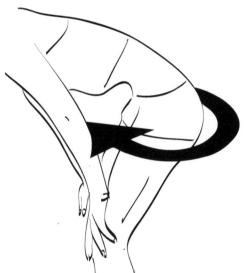

Figure 9.1. Pelvic Circles

Pelvic Floor Massage

Postpartum women can benefit from pelvic floor massage to help realign their bodies after childbirth and improve sexual functioning. Properly done, women report experiencing deeper orgasms. The pelvic floor, with its connections with the abdomen, low back, hips, and legs, has been included in many massage traditions. Rolfing, structural integration, and Hellerwork include pelvic floor work in their efforts

---

1. Dr. Mingdong Li is a teacher and supervisor at Yo San University.

VAGINAL DRYNESS

The drop in hormones and Blood, Yin, and body fluid deficiency after birth can make the vagina drier than normal. It is important to keep the vagina lubricated during intercourse to protect the delicate skin. Aloe vera gel works as an excellent natural water-based lubricant. You can squeeze aloe gel directly into the vagina prior to sex. Some women prefer coconut oil, however, oils degrade latex and the coating of many kegel exercise tools (jade and other crystal eggs are safe).

---

to get the body working as an integrated whole. Some cultures include genital massage to help repair physical trauma and release trapped emotional trauma; such as some Daoist and Tantric traditions. Additionally, there are physical therapists in France and in other countries that specialize in healing the pelvic floor after childbirth. These are distinct from a purely sexual massage whose only purpose is arousal, and are performed on both men and women.

Daoism and Tantra have long traditions of sexual healing. Unfortunately, much of the neo-Tantra communities in the U.S. (and perhaps elsewhere) are corrupted with predatory behavior, guru-worship, and other darkness that threatens to overshadow its light. Both traditional lineage-based Daoism and modern Westernized Daoism have their own share of manipulation, particularly of women students. If you feel drawn to learn more about these practices, just be wary of charismatic figures and always trust your instincts.

If you have suffered vaginal birth trauma or suspect scar tissue formation, I recommend seeing a massage therapist who does rolfing or other bodywork that focuses on correcting the overall structure of the body. They will not work on the genitals, but will release the musculature around it. This can be deep work, both physically and emotionally. Another option is to have your partner do the massage. Mantak Chia has a book on the practice of genital massage or Karsai Nei Tsang.[2] The qigong exercise below is a traditional exercise to regain the waistline and rebalance hormones.

Exercise 9.2. Swimming Dragon Qigong (Figure 9.2)

Women's waists tend to widen in proportion to the rest of the body as female hormones decrease and Spleen Qi weakens. Several seated and standing versions of this exercise exist in different qigong traditions. They involve using a serpentine movement that mobilizes all the joints of the body. My teacher's teacher used this exercise to start her menses again so she could have a child. It also lubricates the joints, increases mobility, narrows the waist, and balances the hormones. Moving slowly allows you to tune into your own energy. Perform 16 repetitions twice a day for maximum benefit.

---

2. Mantak Chi. *Karsai Nei Tsang; Genital Therapeutic Cleansing Massage.* (Chiang Mai: Universal Tao Publications, 2003). Karsai Nei Tsang is offered at the Tao Gardens clinic in Thailand. During a class there a fellow student had been intrigued by the idea. He came back from the experience quite shaken, however, when rather than an erotic experience he instead received quite thorough therapy.

1. Keep feet and palms together for the entire exercise. You will be using your hands to draw a figure 8, crossing the body at the throat, heart, and lower abdomen then back up again.
2. Bring your palms together to the right of the head, face turned to the left, hips sticking out to the left.
3. Cross your hands across your body at throat level to the left side of your body as your face and hips move to the right. Continue the figure 8 motion.
4. Cross your hands across your body at heart level back to the right side as your face and hips move back to the left. Continue the figure 8 motion.
5. Cross your hands across your body at the level of the lower abdomen to the left as your face and hips move to the right.
6. Work back up your body.
7. Perform 16 repetitions.

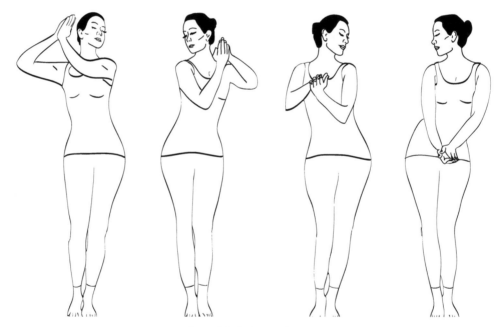

Figure 9.2. Swimming Dragon

The Postpartum Recovery Diet Plan

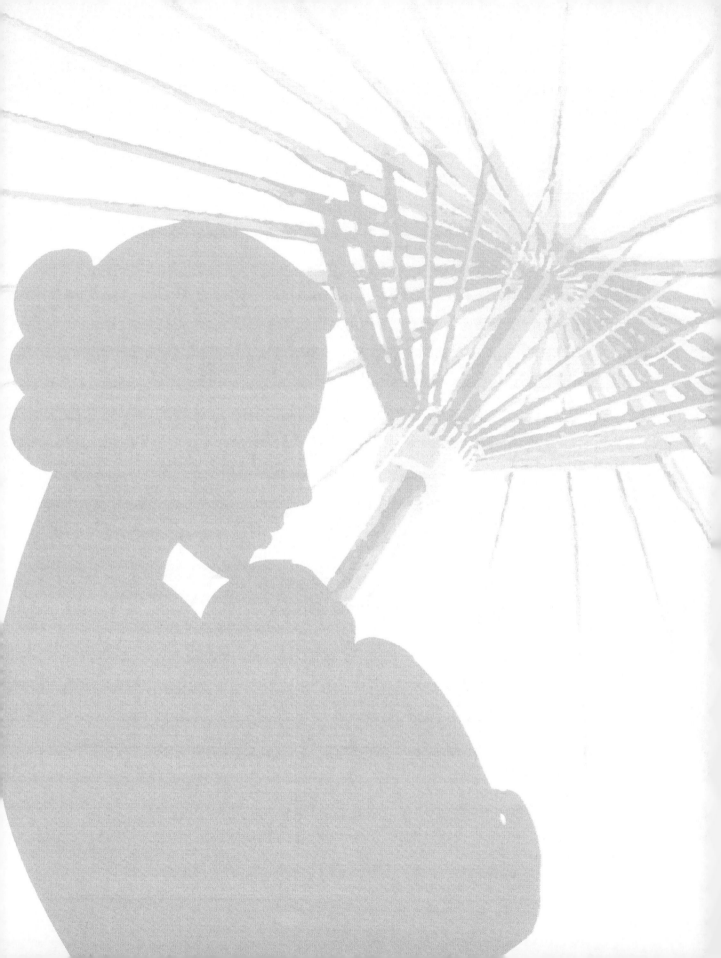

Chapter 10

Ingredients

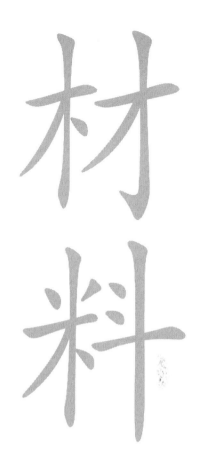

He that takes medicine and neglects diet, wastes the skills of the physician.
Chinese Proverb

Chinese diet therapy, or TCM nutrition, is an essential part of the Postpartum Recovery Program™. In this chapter we will go over the core ingredients that will nourish your body after childbirth and during breastfeeding.

Chinese Superfoods - Food Herbs

Food herbs are Chinese superfoods. These are everyday foods with special properties that can be eaten on a daily basis to strengthen the body and promote longevity.

Disclaimer: "Food herbs" are listed here. These are foods that are used both in herbal formulas and in Chinese diet therapy. Food herbs are generally safe but should still be used with caution by those on medication, particularly blood thinners, and those with serious medical conditions. When in doubt consult your health care professional. If you are a practitioner and want to learn herbal formulas, please see the professional edition of this book[1] or my Postpartum CEU course.[2] Herbs are medicine and require a licensed professional to be used safely. Purchase sulfate-free, organic, herbs and food herbs from reputable distributers.

1. **Black Sesame Seed – Hei Zhi Ma** – tonifies Blood and Jing, moistens dryness, beautifies the hair, and lubricates the intestines. It is used in TCM to treat insufficient breast milk, blurred vision, premature gray hair, dizziness, tinnitus, constipation, and to beautify the skin. Black sesame seed and its oil is a key postpartum food.

2. **Go Ji Berry – Gou Qi Zi** – is a premier longevity tonic that can be used long-term without side effects. It brightens the eyes, nourishes Yin of the Liver, Kidneys, and Lungs. It is used in TCM to treat symptoms such as blurry vision, premature graying hair, soreness of low back and knees, dizziness, infertility, night sweats, dry cough, steaming bones sensations,[3] dry skin, and general anti-aging.[4] Go ji berries are used in many postpartum recovery recipes.

3. **Longan Berry – Long Yan Rou** – is a second longevity tonic that can be used long-term without side effects. It beautifies the skin, tonifies Qi and Blood of the Spleen and Heart, and calms the Shen (spirit or mind). It is very high in iron. Longan berries are used in TCM to treat symptoms like palpitations, difficulty falling and staying asleep, forgetfulness, fatigue, excessive worrying, recovering the mind from studying, emotional sensitivity, physical weakness, shortness of breath, spontaneous sweating, and pallor. Use liberally postpartum.

4. **Mulberry – Sang Shen** – is a third longevity tonic that can be used long-term without side effects. It nourishes Blood and Yin of the Liver and Kidneys, generates body fluids to replenish fluid loss, and lubricates the intestines for deficiency constipation. It is used in TCM to treat dizziness, night sweats, premature graying hair, soreness of low back and knees, tinnitus, and insomnia. Use liberally postpartum.

5. **Hawthorn Berry – Shan Zha** – resolves food stagnation and moves the Blood. It is used in TCM as a digestive (particularly of meat), to treat abdominal bloating and diarrhea, to alleviate abdominal pain postpartum, and to lower serum cholesterol. Caution: hawthorn berry is very sour and can aggravate acid reflux. It can be taken daily in a tea if well-tolerated.

6. **Coix Seeds (Job's Tears) – Yi Yi Ren** – clear Dampness and water retention, clears Heat and pus, tonifies the Spleen, and clears toxicity. Coix seeds gently balance the congesting nature of a high protein diet. They are helpful for intestinal inflammatory disorders as they clear Heat (inflammation), toxicity, and Dampness from the intestines. They are used in TCM to treat a variety of conditions such as edema, loose stools, loss of appetite, acne, tight tendons, joint stiffness and pain, lung or intestinal abscess, and general toxicity. Coix seeds

---

1. Lia Andrews. The Postpartum Recovery Program™; How to Adapt the Ancient Practice of Zuo Yue Zi for Your Patients. (San Diego, Alcyone Press, 2014).

2.www.pacificcenterforlifelonglearning.com.

3. Steaming bone sensation is a symptom that can occur during menopause and some febrile diseases whereby the patient feels like the heat is emanating from their bones.

4. For men, taking a handful of go ji berries daily alleviates symptoms of inflamed prostate such as frequent urination.

are different from pearl barley and are gluten-free. They can be ordered from Asian food markets or Chinese herb shops.

7. **Poria - Fu Ling** - strengthens Spleen Qi, resolves Dampness and Phlegm, and calms the Shen (spirit). It is used in TCM to treat edema, abdominal bloating, accumulations of water or Phlegm, loose stools, fatigue, loss of appetite, insomnia, and palpitations. Poria is excellent postpartum to alleviate water retention.

8. **Red Adzuki Beans – Chi Xiao Dou** - promotes lactation, is diuretic, reduces water retention, moves the Blood and improves circulation. In TCM it is used to treat edema, constipation, to regulate excess weight, and is used topically for bruises and sores. Limit adzuki bean if you are dry or underweight. Postpartum women should eat adzuki bean daily for the first two weeks postpartum.

9. **Black Wood Ear Mushroom – Hei Mu Er** - nourishes Stomach and Lung Yin, soothes the Stomach, moves the Blood, and resolves Phlegm. It is used in TCM to treat dry cough, dry skin, to regulate blood sugar, reduce serum cholesterol, and inhibit tumor formation. Black wood ear mushroom balances the high protein postpartum diet.

10. **White Cloud Mushroom – Bai Mu Er** - nourishes Stomach and Lung Yin and generates body fluids. It is used in TCM to soothe the stomach, calm 5 Heart Heat,[5] to treat dry cough, wrinkles, and thinning or dry skin. It is sometimes called the poor man's bird nest, in reference to its properties as a rejuvenating tonic.

11. **Chinese Red Date (Jujube) – Hong Zao** - tonifies the Spleen and Stomach, tonifies the Blood, calms the Shen (spirit or mind), and protects the Liver. It is used in TCM to treat fatigue, poor appetite, loose stools, pallor, dizziness, blurred vision, amenorrhea,[6] irritability, disturbed sleep, emotional instability, and to harmonize potentially toxic ingredients. Chinese black dates (Da Zao) are the same herb. Black dates are processed differently, have a strong smoky flavor, and are slightly stronger to tonify Blood (red dates are slightly stronger to tonify Qi).[7]

12. **Chinese Yam (Dioscorea) – (Huai) Shan Yao** - tonifies Spleen Qi, and nourishes Stomach, Lung, and Kidney Yin. It is used in TCM to treat leukorrhea,[8] fatigue, poor appetite, loose stools, dry cough, dry skin, soreness of low back and knees, night sweats, frequent urination. Chinese yam helps recover from illness and gently stimulates peristalsis.

13. **Hemp Seed – Huo Ma Ren** - lubricates the intestines to treat constipation. Constipation should be treated quickly postpartum as it can contribute to organ prolapse. It also beautifies the hair to treat hair loss (internally and topically).

14. **Lotus Nut – Lian Zi** – astringes fluids and keeps them from leaking out, and tonifies the Spleen, Heart, and Kidneys. It is used in TCM to treat anxiety, insomnia, palpitations, leukorrhea,[9] and diarrhea. Lotus nuts are added to many of the postpartum recipes.

---

5. Heat on the head, palms, and soles of the feet. A common Yin deficiency symptom that appears with hormonal imbalances postpartum, during menopause, or due to overwork.

6. No menstruation.

7. John Chen. *Chinese Medical Herbology and Pharmacology.* (City of Industry: Art of Medicine Press, Inc., 2001).

8. Pathological vaginal discharge.

9. Pathological vaginal discharge.

Astringents are critical to use in conjunction with tonics in cases of Blood and/or Yin deficiency. As you are building the fluids you need an agent to maintain these fluids in the body. This is observed during severe blood loss. Patients will get excessively thirsty, drink great quantities of water, which runs right through them. If they take astringents and Blood and Yin tonics they are able to hold on to fluids and generate new blood quickly.

Grains

Grains as a general category tonify Qi. Because Qi is weakened postpartum, grains are a key part of the postpartum recovery diet. Be sure to choose organic, GMO-free foods when possible.

1. **Congee** (粥, *zhōu*) – is a thin porridge made most often with rice, but which can be made with any grain. A small amount of grain is cooked with 5-6 times the amount of water for six hours or overnight. Other ingredients are often added to enhance the health effects. This produces a highly digestible food ideal for breakfast and to recover from illness. Plain rice congee tonifies Qi and Blood, and moistens and cools the body. Even Buddha exalted the benefits of congee, claiming congee "confers 10 things on those who eat it: life and beauty, ease and strength. It dispels hunger, thirst, and wind. It cleanses the bladder. It digests food."[10] Postpartum, it promotes the production of healthy breast milk and should be eaten first thing in the morning. During the month after birth, congee is traditionally made with sweet rice, however I prefer using 1 part jasmine rice to 1 part sweet rice.

2. **Rice** – tonifies Qi, soothes the Stomach to treat fatigue, diarrhea, and irritability, and protects the body from harsh herbs. White rice has a neutral thermal temperature and is considered the ideal food for convalescence and those with weakened digestion. Sweet rice (or glutinous rice) has a stronger action to strengthen Qi, is higher in protein, warms the body, helps check spontaneous sweating, and is often recommended for postpartum women. Contrary to the name, it is safe for gluten-free diets, like all rice. Sweet rice can create Phlegm when eaten in excess. Basmati rice is the most aromatic and best for overweight, stagnant, Damp individuals. Brown rice is more heating and harder to digest than white rice, but high in B vitamins. Soak eight hours prior to cooking to increase digestibility as you would legumes. Black glutinous rice is strongest to tonify Blood and also strengthens Kidney Yin.

3. **Oats** – are warming, moistening, tonify Qi, and are high in protein.

4. **Barley** – is cooling, tonifies Qi and Blood, and nourishes Yin.

5. **Millet** – is cooling, tonifies Qi and Yin, and moistens dryness.

6. **Buckwheat** – is neutral and high in protein. Roasted buckwheat (kasha) dries Dampness.

7. **Wheat** – is cooling, tonifies Qi, nourishes Yin, calms the Shen (spirit or mind), and promotes weight gain for the underweight. Wheat has been heavily modified in the last century and increasing numbers of people are sensitive to it. Buy non-GMO wheat

---

10. Shakyamuni Buddha, Makavagga, Vinanaya Pitaka (Book of the Discipline), trans. By I. B. Harner, London, 1951, Vol. IV, p.302.

products or older wheat strains such as Kamut or spelt. Wholegrain sprouted wheat bread is tolerated well by some who cannot eat refined wheat flour products. Bulghur wheat is an excellent protein source.

8. **Quinoa** – is warming, tonifies Qi and Kidney Yang, and is very high in protein.
9. **Corn** – is neutral, helps regulate digestion, and strengthens the Kidneys. Whole cornmeal cooked with figs, dates, or prunes (for good measure) is an excellent antidote to constipation.

Vegetables

Vegetables as a group clear excesses from the body. Raw vegetables are more cooling and clearing and best suited to excess and robust individuals. Cooked vegetables are more neutral and appropriate for weaker conditions. Unless you run hot, eat mostly cooked vegetables postpartum. Fermenting vegetables also renders them more digestible and are fine in small amounts postpartum. Avoid raw vegetables and fruits particularly during the first two weeks postpartum, unless otherwise advised by your acupuncturist or you are suffering from Heat signs (see page 43).

1. **Shitake Mushroom** – moves the Blood, clears Phlegm-Damp from the body, and boosts immunity. It helps reduce cholesterol and fat from the body. All mushrooms have this effect to a greater or lesser degrees. The clearing nature of shitake mushroom balances the rich, high protein postpartum recovery diet.
2. **Daikon Radish** – resolves Phlegm-Dampness, clears Heat, and detoxifies the body (especially the Lungs and intestines). Like shitake mushroom, daikon radish balances a rich, high protein diet. Note: daikon radish is very mild in taste but it is quite stinky, unless freshly cut, particularly if pickled. When cooked the smell is harmonized with the other ingredients.
3. **Dark Leafy Greens** – nourish Blood and Yin, and clear excess particularly of the Liver and Gallbladder system. **Spinach** is an excellent blood builder, is cooling, and laxative. **Kale, collard greens**, and **swiss chard** are also high in chlorophyll and strong blood builders. The more bitter the greens, the more cooling, dispersing, and detoxifying they are. **Mustard greens** are warm and resolve Phlegm-Damp. **Watercress** is cooling, promotes urination, and moves Blood. Note: spinach, Swiss chard, beet greens, collards are high in oxalate and excess consumption may inhibit calcium absorption and contribute to Kidney stone formation.
4. **Yam and Sweet Potato** - tonify Qi and Blood, nourish Yin, and promote breast milk production. They benefit the eyes.
5. **Carrot** – tonifies Qi and Blood, regulates the Liver to balance hormones, and benefits the eyes.
6. **Beet** – nourishes Blood and regulates the Liver to help balance hormones.

Fruit

Eat fruit sparingly for the first two weeks, with the exception of cooked green papaya and the food herbs mentioned above. Fruit is more cooling than vegetables and should be cooked during the first two weeks postpartum. After the first two weeks, eat 1-2 servings of fruit each day. Certain fruits are very effective for treating constipation such as prune, banana, and apricot.

1. **Green Papaya (unripe red or yellow papaya)** – is a traditional food to boost breast milk production and promote lactation. Papaya is also rich in enzymes, dispels parasites,[11] and resolves Phlegm-Damp. Include green and ripe papaya frequently in the diet, in soups and salads.
2. **Berries (blueberry, strawberry, raspberry, mulberry)** – generally tonify Liver Blood and nourish Kidney Yin. Add them to congee or hot cereals for breakfast.

Animal Products & Protein-Rich Foods

Animal products are the strongest foods to build Qi and Blood, which is why they figure so centrally in the postpartum recovery diet. The postpartum month is the most challenging time for a woman to be vegan and she will need to rely more on superfoods and herbal formulas to strengthen her. Animal products raise the biggest issues in terms of ethics and food safety. Be sure to choose organic, humanely raised animal products. In this list are also popular meat substitutes.

1. **Eggs** – are a strong and easily digestible Qi and Blood tonic. Traditionally, they are boiled and soaked in vinegar for one month prior to childbirth, then eaten daily for two weeks. They are also cooked with vinegar and pork trotters (see Pork Trotter's & Peanut Soup on page 213). Eat eggs frequently during the postpartum month.
2. **Milk and Cheese** – nourish Blood and Yin, are a great source of protein and calcium, but tend to produce Phlegm-Damp. Goat's milk is more Yang in nature, and less likely to cause Dampness. Use milk and cheese sparingly, with the exception of kefir.

> **THE POWER OF LIVER**
> Our dog Lola suffered a severe internal hemorrhage and lost so much blood the vet said she would not make it through the night. When Lola got home she was drinking water constantly and urinating everything she drank almost immediately. I made her Liver Congee #1 (page 162) which contains lotus nuts, along with Yunnan Baiyao capsules and Si Wu Tang teapills, a Blood tonifying formula. She stopped the excessive thirst and urination within an hour. One week later her tongue was back to a healthy pink and she was full of energy. The vet confirmed a few weeks later her blood was back to normal.

---

11. This antiparasitic action is increased by soaking green papaya in vinegar. Paul Pirchford, *Healing with Whole Foods; Ancient Tradition and Modern Nutrition.* (Berkeley: North Atlantic Books, 1993).

3. **Liver** – is the strongest food to build Liver Blood, benefits the eyes, and some claim it has a moving and detoxifying effect.[12] Traditionally, pork liver is used postpartum, due to its neutral thermal temperature and ability to nourish Kidney Yin, however it is the most bitter-tasting of the livers. Chicken liver is heating but tastier. Beef liver is also neutral and sits between chicken and pork in taste. Many are concerned about the safety of liver. A 2004 study showed, however, that the liver was no more toxic than lean meat of the same animal, though kidney is markedly more toxic.[13] As with all meat, be sure to eat organic, humanely raised liver. Soak liver in lime or lemon juice, vinegar, or milk for 30 minutes prior to cooking to fully clean it and improve its taste. Traditionally, liver is eaten daily for the first week postpartum to quickly replenish blood loss.[14]

4. **Kidneys** – strengthens the Kidneys, low back and knees, and helps contract the uterus. For this reason, it is traditionally eaten daily during the second week postpartum.[15] Again, pork kidneys are traditionally eaten, and again these are the least palatable. Lamb or beef kidneys taste better and are easier to come by in the U.S. Kidneys are riskier to eat in terms of toxicity and must be thoroughly cleaned prior to cooking. If you choose to eat them you must find a clean source and watch a YouTube video on proper cleaning. Cut the kidney in half, and cut out the ureters (all the white membranes). Cooking scissors work well for this. Then soak in lime or lemon juice for 30 minutes prior to cooking.

5. **Chicken** – tonifies Qi and Jing and promotes lactation. Traditionally, chicken is eaten daily during the third, fourth, and fifth weeks postpartum, and three times a week as long as the mother is breastfeeding.[16] Black silkie chickens (烏骨雞, wū gǔ jī, literally "black-boned chicken") are considered the strongest to tonify Blood.

6. **Pork Trotters (Pig's Feet)** – tonifies Qi and Blood, nourishes Kidney Yin, and promotes healthy breast milk. It combines the calcium and bone-building effects of bone broth with added collagen to strengthen joints and ligaments. Pork trotter soup includes peanuts and Chinese herbs to form the quintessential breast milk-promoting recipe. High collagen foods also help rehabilitate the pelvic floor after vaginal delivery and the abdomen after C-section.

7. **Fish** – is an easily digestible protein source which strengthens Qi, moistens dryness, and dissolves obstruction. **Carp** is frequently used postpartum as it reduces edema and promotes lactation, particularly when paired with tofu. Traditionally, during the first week postpartum women eat **threadfin fish** (烏仔魚, wū zǐ yú, Eleutheronema rhadinum) and **yellow croaker** (黃花魚, huáng huā yú, Larimichthys crocea), as they are considered easier to digest. Women who have had a C-section are given **perch** (鱸魚, lú yú, Perca fluviatilis)

---

12. Shuqi Zhuang. *Postpartum Recovery Program; a Manual of Rules and Recipes for the Postpartum Woman.* (Taiwan: Guang He Chu Ban She, 2005). ISBN 9578807015

13. Irfana Mariam, Shehla Iqbal, and Saeed Ahmad Nagra, "Distribution of Some Trace and Macrominerals in Beef, Mutton, and Poultry," International Journal of Agriculture & Biology (2004), 1560-8530/06-5-816-820, www.ijab.org

14. Shuqi Zhuang. *Postpartum Recovery Program; a Manual of Rules and Recipes for the Postpartum Woman.* (Taiwan: Guang He Chu Ban She, 2005). ISBN 9578807015

15. Ibid.

16. Ibid.

during the third-fifth weeks to promote wound healing.[17] Cod, halibut, and sea bass are other common choices. Choose fish that you enjoy.

8. **Seitan** – also known as "wheat meat," is wheat gluten that has been extracted from wheat flour. It is very high in protein. However, it has a cold thermal temperature making it harder to digest and prone to generating Dampness. It is best for those who run hot. For postpartum women be sure to balance its cold nature by cooking thoroughly with warming spices.

9. **Tofu** – or bean curd, is coagulated soybean milk. It is high in protein and calcium, and moistens dryness. It is available in extra firm, firm, and soft/silken forms. Tofu is cold in nature, hard on digestion, and tends to create Dampness. It is best for those who run hot and dry, particularly menopausal women. For postpartum women be sure to balance its cold nature by cooking thoroughly with warming spices. Tofu skin or bean curd skin (腐皮, fǔ pí) is made by boiling soy milk and skimming the curd off the top. Tofu skin provides an excellent texture and mild taste for stir fries and soups.

10. **Tempeh** – is fermented soybeans mixture with other grains or legumes. It has the same benefits and drawbacks as seitan and tofu. Cook with warming spices.

Miscellaneous

1. **Salt** – avoid using salt to flavor foods. It will increase water retention and slow the process of discharging excess fluids from the body. A trick to minimize salt is to make recipes without salt and add as little as you can when you sit down to eat. You will end up using less salt.

2. **Ginger (browned)** – cook most of your food with browned ginger. That is, sauté the ginger until it develops a crunchy brown layer on both sides. Do not blacken, however. Charred herbs are used to stop bleeding, and we do not want to interrupt the discharge of lochia. The preparation of ginger is very important. Fresh ginger goes to the Lungs and Stomach. Charred ginger astringes menstrual blood. Dried ginger goes to the Stomach and Spleen, warming digestion. Browned ginger goes to the uterus, warming it, and facilitates the passage of menses and lochia.

3. **Garlic** – is an extremely heating substance. Avoid it if there are Yin deficiency or Heat signs such as feeling hot, hot flashes, acne, mastitis, yellow vaginal discharge, irritability, mouth sores, night sweats, or insomnia. However if you run cold, garlic effectively warms up the body. A little goes a long way. Limit yourself to ½ to 1 small clove of garlic in recipes.

4. **Black Sesame Oil** – use cold pressed, organic black sesame oil as your main cooking oil. Like black sesame seeds, it lubricates the intestines facilitating bowel movements, tonifies Qi and Blood to recover strength, and protects against Wind Invasion by boosting immunity. It is also a versatile cooking oil.

5. **Chinese Rice Wine** – is not sake, which is more like rice beer. Rice wine has an alcohol

---

17. Shuqi Zhuang. *Postpartum Recovery Program; a Manual of Rules and Recipes for the Postpartum Woman.* (Taiwan: Guang He Chu Ban She, 2005). ISBN 9578807015

content of 18%–25%; higher than beer, sake, or grape wine. Rice wine warms the body and moves stagnant Blood, performing two necessary actions postpartum. Add ¼ - ½ cup to soups and stews. If unavailable, substitute with dry sherry. Many modern Taiwanese women use special rice wine that has had most of its alcohol content removed.[18]

6. **Placenta** – is the medicinal substance closest to Jing we can consume. The placenta contains hormones and nutrients that can help speed postpartum recovery. It was traditionally eaten by postpartum mothers to help them recover hormonal balance. Placenta encapsulation is a modern take on an old practice, and is performed by practitioners trained in placenta encapsulation. This is a sanitary method by which the placenta is washed, dehydrated, and put into capsules to be taken throughout the first postpartum month.[19] I recommend finding someone who is trained in a safe method of doing this or becoming trained yourself (though you will be in no condition to prepare your placenta after giving birth). You will also need to make special arrangements during delivery to save your placenta and bring a cooler to store it. Note: make sure that only powdered placenta is in the capsules, not additional herbs, unless given by a TCM herbalist. Additional herbs are best taken separately. Placenta is a warming substance and may need to be taken with other herbs to balance it (Placenta Encapsulation on page 245).[20]

7. **Seaweed** – all types of seaweed are cooling and moistening, regulate water metabolism, detoxify the lymphatic system, dissolve Phlegm, and soften hardness. Seaweed treats every type of swelling: inflammation, nodules, tumors, edema, excess weight, and cystic acne. It is also nutrient-dense and treats constipation. Use seaweed cautiously during postpartum as it has a cooling thermal temperature, however it is a gentle remedy for constipation or any inflammatory symptoms that arise. **Kelp (kombu)** seaweed has the strongest action and is most often used in medicine and food therapy.

8. **Algae** – nourishes Blood. Though it is cooling in nature, it is an excellent blood builder for vegans. Postpartum take chlorella or spirulina tablets daily with warm water.

9. **Probiotics** – are beneficial bacteria that assist in the digestive process. Spleen Qi is weakened postpartum, meaning digestion is weaker. It is a good idea to take probiotics and digestive enzyme supplements or consume homemade probiotics, like kefir.

10. **Unrefined Brown Sugar (muscovado, molasses sugar)** – is the traditionally used sweetener chosen due to its warming thermal nature. It moves and nourishes Blood. Use sparingly, as the modern diet typically has too much sugar in it.

11. **Peanuts** – nourish Qi, Blood, and Yin, and promote lactation. They are used in TCM

---

18. A popular brand is 廣和坐月子水 Guang He Zuo Yue Zi Shui – literally "Great Harmony Postpartum Recovery Water." It can be purchased at www.JingMommy.com.

19. The method I have heard most used is: Make arrangements ahead of time with the hospital to bring your placenta home with you. You will want to bring it home in a cooler on ice and either prepare it immediately or store it in the freezer until you are ready to use it. To process, rinse the placenta and cut into small pieces, removing the veins. Steam the pieces until they are soft. Then put the pieces in a dehydrating machine to dry out the placenta until it became brittle. Crush the dehydrated pieces into fine powder form. You can use an encapsulation machine to put the powder into capsules.

20. Dosage recommendations vary and may need to be modified for the individual as placenta is warming and strongly tonifying. A typical dosage schedule is as follows: **Days 1 – 3:** Take 2 capsules 3 times per day (six total), with meals. **Days 4 – 14:** Take 2 capsules 2 times per day (four total), with meals. **Days 14 and beyond:** Take 2 capsules 1 time per day with a meal until you run out.

to treat insufficient lactation due to deficiency. Eaten in excess they can cause Phlegm-Dampness.

Liquids

Drink only warm drinks and soups. You can choose from Red Date Tea, Adzuki Bean Tea, Postpartum Tea, etc.

Property	Warming	Move Blood	Tonify Qi & Blood	Nourish Kidney	Promote Lactation	Detoxify
Foods	Rice wine, ginger, garlic, beef, chicken, lamb.	Rice wine, ginger (browned), liver, black wood ear fungus, hawthorn berry, sweet rice, vinegar.	Liver, longan berry, red date, Chinese yam, go ji berry, congee, eggs, chicken, sweet rice.	Black sesame seed and oil, placenta, Chinese yam, go ji berry, kidney.	Peanut, pork trotters, carp and tofu, black sesame seed, green papaya, adzuki bean.	Coix seeds, adzuki bean, shitake mushroom, seaweed, mung bean, black wood ear fungus, daikon radish, tea, hawthorn berry.

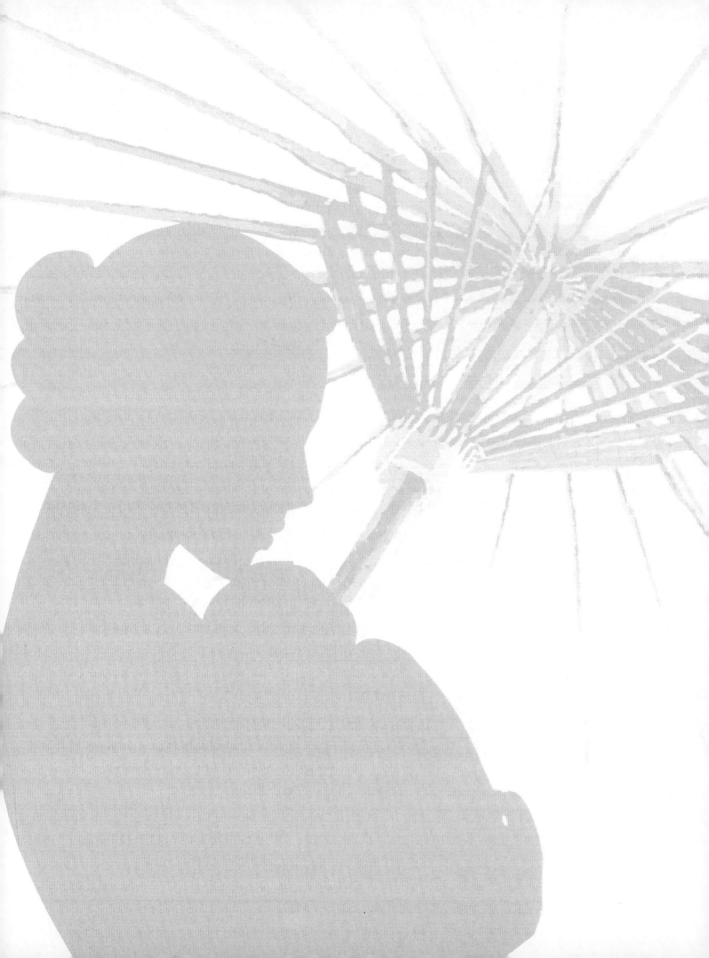

Chapter 11
Meal Plans

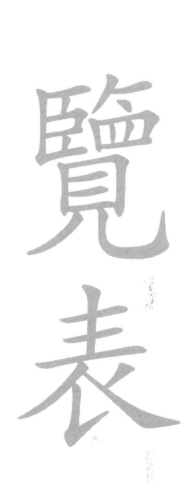

Diet is an essential piece of the Postpartum Recovery Program™. This chapter will show there are many ways to create a meal plan that will rebuild your body.

Preparation Options

There are a few options for getting your postpartum meals. If you are extremely lucky, you will have a family member, friend, or hired help to prepare meals for you. Most women do not have this option, however. If you live close to a Chinese or Taiwanese immigrant community, you can arrange for a postpartum meal delivery service (Postpartum Care on page 245). This is the easiest and most expensive option. These services often offer the option to pick up the meals frozen at a reduced price.

You can also prepare the recipes yourself ahead of time and freeze. This is the most economical and allows you to cook for your taste. I recommend freezing the recipes in the proper portions and organizing them by stage so you can easily take them out and heat them each day. You might need to purchase a small freezer for this.

Do Not Overeat

You need to eat adequately to recover postpartum, especially if you are breastfeeding. However, be careful not to overdo it. Water retention easily converts to fat at this time.

Vegetarian Options

Pregnancy, breastfeeding, and menstruation are the most challenging times to forgo animal products. Extra effort must be made to tonify the Blood. Besides diet, you will need to rely more heavily on herbal formulas given by a TCM herbalist. See the Pescatarian Meal Plan (page 141) and Vegan Meal Plan (page 145). Adding fish and eggs to the diet greatly improves tonification.

Taste

The traditional diet is bland and easy to digest. Make yourself comfortable. Feel free to modify the diet to your taste, like substituting other grains for rice. However, be sure to keep the bulk of the diet cooked and protein-rich. Warming spices, such as ginger, white pepper, and cardamom, are recommended for most postpartum women to protect the body from Cold and support passage of the lochia. Avoid spices if the climate is hot or if you are feeling warm, crave cold drinks, or are experiencing dryness.

Breakfast Options

The natural daily cycle is that Yang is strongest in the morning and weakest in the evening. If we are to follow this cycle we should eat out biggest and most complicated meals for breakfast and lunch. Breakfast should consist of well-cooked grains, vegetables, and protein. If constipation is an issue, include one or more of these ingredients daily: black sesame seed or oil, hemp seed, banana, prune, apricot, spinach, and beet.

Lunch Options

Eat red adzuki beans daily for the first two weeks, as a tea, soup, over rice, or as dessert. During the first week, try to incorporate organic liver. For the more adventurous, during the second week, try to incorporate organic kidney. And for the third, fourth, and fifth weeks include organic chicken. Fish is also an excellent source of protein. If you cannot stomach organ meats, substitute with a rare steak.

Dinner Options

Dinner should be the simplest and lightest meal of the day. Aim to finish dinner by 7pm. I recommend a vegetable-based soup or stew.

Chinese Herbs

A TCM herbalist can give herbs to prevent or resolve many postpartum symptoms. Appropriate herbs will also build strength and vitality, so that you recover quickly and completely from childbirth. Note: a Western herbalist will not be familiar with the unique and intricate system of Chinese herbs. Be sure to find a practitioner who is board certified in Chinese herbal medicine.[1]

Beverages

Sip warm and herbal teas throughout the day. There are several teas that are helpful postpartum, such as Red Date Tea and Postpartum Tea,

Next are example meal plans.

---

1. Professional titles vary from state to state and internationally. For example, the state of California requires extensive herbal knowledge to become a licensed acupuncturist (L.Ac.), though it may not be obvious in the title. Other states may separate acupuncture and herbal practice, or not cover herbal medicine at all. To check the regulations and licensing for your state please see www.Acufinder.com/Acupuncture+Laws

Basic Meal Plan

Table 11.1 shows the basic outline for the Postpartum Recovery Meal Plan™. The traditional postpartum diet is bland and repetitive; true convalescent food. This makes it easy to digest, and also easy to plan for. You are free to make the meal plan as simple or as exciting as you like. There are sample meal plans on the next few pages for different diets. There is also an extensive recipe list at the end of this book to inspire your creativity.

Stage 1 - Week 1

Treatment Principle: Detoxify the body and discharge lochia.

The focus of the first week is to gently discharge from the body the lochia and any residual contents from the womb. Water retention needs to be efficiently cleared as well. However, the body is also at its weakest, so extra care must be taken to conserve Qi and Blood.

Stage 2 - Week 2

Treatment Principle: Contract the internal organs, uterus, and pelvic cavity.

After much of the excesses have been discharged from the body, the focus of the second week is to contract everything back to its normal size.

Stage 3 - Weeks 3-4 (&5)

Treatment Principle: Nourish, supplement, and renew strength.

After two weeks the body has been cleared of toxins enough to focus primarily on tonifying. Repeat the recipes as necessary for the fifth week.

Table 11.1. Basic Meal Plan

	Week 1	Week 2	Week 3-4 (&5)
Breakfast	Congee Eggs or Vegetarian Protein Serving of vegetables		
Empty Stomach Before Lunch	Herbal tea from TCM herbalist		
Lunch	Liver, Steak, or Vegetarian Protein Rice or other Grain Serving of Vegetables	Kidney, Steak, or Vegetarian Protein Rice or other Grain Serving of Vegetables	Chicken, Steak, or Vegetarian Protein Rice or other Grain Serving of Vegetables
Empty Stomach Before Dinner	Herbal tea from TCM herbalist		
Dinner	Fish Soup or Vegetarian Soup		Fish Soup or Vegetarian Soup Lactation-Promoting Soup 1-3 times a week if breastfeeding
Snacks	Red Adzuki Bean Tea (page 159) or Sweet Adzuki Bean Soup (page 178)		Serving of Fruit
Drinks (Throughout the Day)	Red Date Tea (page 157) Postpartum Tea (page 158)		Date and White Cloud Tea (page 160) Red Adzuki Bean Tea (page 159)

Simplified Omnivore Meal Plan

The following is an example of a simple meal plan. It is repetitive but easy to plan for. If you cannot palate organ meats, substitute fish or a rare steak. Beef is considered too heating and difficult to digest for the first two weeks postpartum according to traditional postpartum theory. However, beef strongly tonifies Qi and Blood, making it a powerful substitute for liver. You should also include probiotics, such as kefir water, in your daily diet to strengthen digestion.

Stage 1 - Week 1

Treatment Principle: Detoxify the body and discharge lochia.

The focus of the first week is to gently discharge from the body the lochia and any residual contents from the womb. Water retention needs to be efficiently cleared as well. However, the body is also at its weakest, so extra care must be taken to conserve Qi and Blood.

Stage 2 - Week 2

Treatment Principle: Contract the internal organs, uterus, and pelvic cavity.

After much of the excesses have been discharged from the body, the focus of the second week is to contract everything back to its normal size.

Stage 3 - Weeks 3-4 (&5)

Treatment Principle: Nourish, supplement, and renew strength.

After two weeks the body has been cleared of toxins enough to focus primarily on tonifying. Repeat the recipes as necessary for the fifth week.

Table 11.2. Sample Simplified Meal Plan Week 1

	Breakfast	**Tea**	**Lunch**	**Tea**	**Dinner**
Day 1	Liver Congee #2 (page 163) Placenta capsules	Red Date Tea (page 157) Postpartum Tea (page 158) Herbal tea from TCM herbalist	Liver Congee #2 (page 163) Placenta capsules	Red Date Tea (page 157) Postpartum Tea (page 158) Herbal tea from TCM herbalist	Fish and Carrot Soup (page 210) Red Adzuki Bean Tea (page 159) Placenta capsules
Day 2					
Day 3					
Day 4	Water Reducing Congee (page 165) Go Ji Eggs (page 171) Steamed vegetables Placenta capsules		Simple Liver & Onions (page 185) Yi Ren Rice (page 180) Steamed vegetables		Coconut Fish Soup (page 210) Red Adzuki Bean Tea (page 159) Placenta capsules
Day 5			Liver Ragu (page 187)		
Day 6			Simple Liver & Onions (page 185) Yi Ren Rice (page 180) Steamed vegetables		Carp and Tofu Soup (page 211) Red Adzuki Bean Tea (page 159) Placenta capsules
Day 7			Liver Ragu (page 187)		

Table 11.3. Sample Simplified Meal Plan Week 2

	Breakfast	Tea	Lunch	Tea	Dinner
Day 8	Water Reducing Congee (page 165) Go Ji Eggs (page 171) Steamed vegetables Placenta capsules	Postpartum Tea (page 158) Herbal tea from TCM herbalist	Liver with Potatoes (page 190) Sautéed greens	Postpartum Tea (page 158) Herbal tea from TCM herbalist	Carp and Tofu Soup (page 211) Red Adzuki Bean Tea (page 159) Placenta capsules
Day 9			Simple Liver & Onions (page 185) Stir-Fried Sticky Rice (page 181) Steamed asparagus		
Day 10	Cereal Milk (page 167) Beijing Eggs (page 172) Sautéed greens Placenta capsules		Beef & Kidney Stroganoff (page 197) Yi Ren Rice (page 180) Steamed vegetables		Fish and Carrot Soup (page 210) Red Adzuki Bean Tea (page 159) Placenta capsules
Day 11					
Day 12	Water Reducing Congee (page 165) Green Tea Eggs (page 172) Steamed vegetables Placenta capsules		Steak & Kidney Pie (page 195)		Carp and Green Papaya Soup (page 212) Red Adzuki Bean Tea (page 159) Placenta capsules
Day 13					
Day 14	Cereal Milk (page 167) Beijing Eggs (page 172) Sautéed greens Placenta capsules		Devilled Kidneys on Toast (page 198) Sautéed greens		Fish and Carrot Soup (page 210) Red Adzuki Bean Tea (page 159) Placenta capsules

Table 11.4. Sample Simplified Meal Plan Weeks 3-4 (&5)

	Breakfast	Tea	Lunch	Tea	Dinner
Day 15/22	Canja de Galinha (page 164)	Date and White Cloud Tea (page 160) Red Adzuki Bean Tea (page 159) Herbal tea from TCM herbalist	Rare steak Yi Ren Rice (page 180) Steamed vegetables	Date and White Cloud Tea (page 160) Red Adzuki Bean Tea (page 159) Herbal tea from TCM herbalist	Fish and Carrot Soup (page 210) Placenta capsules
Day 16/23			Sautéed Ginger Chicken (page 199) Stir-Fried Sticky Rice (page 181) Steamed vegetables		
Day 17/24					Pork Trotter's & Peanut Soup (page 213) Placenta capsules
Day 18/25			Calamondin Roast Chicken (page 200) Yi Ren Rice (page 180) Steamed vegetables		
Day 19/26					Carp and Green Papaya Soup (page 212) Placenta capsules
Day 20/27			Sautéed Ginger Chicken (page 199) Yi Ren Rice (page 180) Steamed vegetables		
Day 21/28					Fish and Carrot Soup (page 210) Placenta capsules

Varied Omnivore Meal Plan

In this next meal plan, I have maintained the spirit, and key ingredients, of the traditional Taiwanese plan, while showing an example of how this can be adapted to suit Western tastes. The diet is more neutral in thermal temperature because most Westerners run hotter (i.e. are more inflamed). Thus alcohol and sugar are minimized, and more vegetables are added. If you cannot palate organ meats, substitute eggs for breakfast and a rare steak for lunch. Beef is considered too heating and difficult to digest for the first two weeks postpartum according to traditional postpartum theory. However, beef strongly tonifies Qi and Blood, making it a powerful substitute for liver. You should also include probiotics, such as kefir water, in your daily diet to strengthen digestion.

Stage 1 - Week 1

Treatment Principle: Detoxify the body and discharge lochia.

The focus of the first week is to gently discharge from the body the lochia and any residual contents from the womb. Water retention needs to be efficiently cleared as well. However, the body is also at its weakest, so extra care must be taken to conserve Qi and Blood.

Stage 2 - Week 2

Treatment Principle: Contract the internal organs, uterus, and pelvic cavity.

After much of the excesses have been discharged from the body, the focus of the second week is to contract everything back to its normal size.

Stage 3 - Weeks 3-4 (&5)

Treatment Principle: Nourish, supplement, and renew strength.

After two weeks the body has been cleared of toxins enough to focus primarily on tonifying. Repeat the recipes as necessary for the fifth week.

Table 11.5. Sample Omnivore Meal Plan Week 1

	Breakfast	Tea	Lunch	Tea	Dinner
Day 1	Liver Congee #2 (page 163) Placenta capsules	Red Date Tea (page 157) Postpartum Tea (page 158) Herbal tea from TCM herbalist	Liver Congee #2 (page 163) Placenta capsules	Red Date Tea (page 157) Postpartum Tea (page 158) Herbal tea from TCM herbalist	Fish and Carrot Soup (page 210) Red Adzuki Bean Tea (page 159) Placenta capsules
Day 2					
Day 3	Water Reducing Congee (page 165) Go Ji Eggs (page 171) Steamed carrots Placenta capsules		Liver Ragu (page 187) Placenta capsules		Coconut Fish Soup (page 210) Red Adzuki Bean Tea (page 159) Placenta capsules
Day 4	Cereal Milk (page 167) Beijing Eggs (page 172) Sautéed greens Placenta capsules		Simple Liver & Onions (page 185) Yi Ren Rice (page 180) Steamed asparagus		Carp and Tofu Soup (page 211) Red Adzuki Bean Tea (page 159) Placenta capsules
Day 5	Water Reducing Congee (page 165) Go Ji Eggs (page 171) Steamed beets Placenta capsules		Liver Laab (page 189) Yi Ren Rice (page 180)		Coconut Fish Soup (page 210) Red Adzuki Bean Tea (page 159) Placenta capsules
Day 6	Water Reducing Congee (page 165) Green Tea Eggs (page 172) Steamed carrots Placenta capsules		Pirão de Fígado (page 192) Sautéed Eggplant (page 183)		Fish and Carrot Soup (page 210) Red Adzuki Bean Tea (page 159) Placenta capsules
Day 7	Cereal Milk (page 167) Beijing Eggs (page 172) Sautéed greens Placenta capsules		Liver with Wine Sauce (page 191) Yi Ren Rice (page 180) Steamed asparagus		Carp and Green Papaya Soup (page 212) Red Adzuki Bean Tea (page 159) Placenta capsules

Table 11.6. Sample Omnivore Meal Plan Week 2

	Breakfast	Tea	Lunch	Tea	Dinner
Day 8	Water Reducing Congee (page 165) Go Ji Eggs (page 171) Steamed vegetables Placenta capsules	Postpartum Tea (page 158) Herbal tea from TCM herbalist	Liver with Potatoes (page 190) Sautéed greens	Postpartum Tea (page 158) Herbal tea from TCM herbalist	Carp and Tofu Soup (page 211) Red Adzuki Bean Tea (page 159) Placenta capsules
Day 9	Water Reducing Congee (page 165) Green Tea Eggs (page 172) Sautéed eggplant Placenta capsules		Simple Liver & Onions (page 185) Stir-Fried Sticky Rice (page 181) Steamed asparagus		Coconut Fish Soup (page 210) Red Adzuki Bean Tea (page 159) Placenta capsules
Day 10	Cornmeal Congee (page 169) Go Ji Eggs (page 171) Steamed vegetables Placenta capsules		Beef & Kidney Stroganoff (page 197) Yi Ren Rice (page 180)		Fish and Carrot Soup (page 210) Red Adzuki Bean Tea (page 159) Placenta capsules
Day 11	Cereal Milk (page 167) Beijing Eggs (page 172) Sautéed greens Placenta capsules		Steak & Kidney Pie (page 195)		Carp and Green Papaya Soup (page 212) Red Adzuki Bean Tea (page 159) Placenta capsules
Day 12	Water Reducing Congee (page 165) Green Tea Eggs (page 172) Steamed vegetables Placenta capsules		Steak & Kidney Pie (page 195)		Carp and Tofu Soup (page 211) Red Adzuki Bean Tea (page 159) Placenta capsules
Day 13	Cereal Milk (page 167) Beijing Eggs (page 172) Sautéed greens Placenta capsules		Pirão de Rim (page 196) Steamed asparagus		Coconut Fish Soup (page 210) Red Adzuki Bean Tea (page 159) Placenta capsules
Day 14	Water Reducing Congee (page 165) Go Ji Eggs (page 171) Steamed vegetables Placenta capsules		Devilled Kidneys on Toast (page 198) Sautéed greens		Fish and Carrot Soup (page 210) Red Adzuki Bean Tea (page 159) Placenta capsules

Table 11.7. Sample Omnivore Meal Plan Week 3

	Breakfast	Tea	Lunch	Tea	Dinner
Day 15	Canja de Galinha (page 164)	Date and White Cloud Tea (page 160) Red Adzuki Bean Tea (page 159) Herbal tea from TCM herbalist	Rare steak Yi Ren Rice (page 180) Steamed vegetables	Date and White Cloud Tea (page 160) Red Adzuki Bean Tea (page 159) Herbal tea from TCM herbalist	Fish and Carrot Soup (page 210) Placenta capsules
Day 16			Calamondin Roast Chicken (page 200) Yi Ren Rice (page 180) Steamed vegetables		Carp and Tofu Soup (page 211) Placenta capsules
Day 17			Sautéed Ginger Chicken (page 199) Yi Ren Rice (page 180) Steamed vegetables		Pork Trotter's & Peanut Soup (page 213) Placenta capsules
Day 18			Rare steak Yi Ren Rice (page 180) Steamed vegetables		Fish and Carrot Soup (page 210) Placenta capsules
Day 19			Sautéed Ginger Chicken (page 199) Yi Ren Rice (page 180) Steamed vegetables		Pork Trotter's & Peanut Soup (page 213) Placenta capsules
Day 20			Calamondin Roast Chicken (page 200) Yi Ren Rice (page 180) Steamed vegetables		Carp and Green Papaya Soup (page 212) Placenta capsules
Day 21			Sautéed Ginger Chicken (page 199) Yi Ren Rice (page 180) Steamed vegetables		Pork Trotter's & Peanut Soup (page 213) Placenta capsules

Table 11.8. Sample Omnivore Meal Plan Week 4

	Breakfast	Tea	Lunch	Tea	Dinner
Day 22	Canja de Galinha (page 164)	Date and White Cloud Tea (page 160) Red Adzuki Bean Tea (page 159) Herbal tea from TCM herbalist	Rare steak Yi Ren Rice (page 180) Steamed vegetables	Date and White Cloud Tea (page 160) Red Adzuki Bean Tea (page 159) Herbal tea from TCM herbalist	Fish and Carrot Soup (page 210)
Day 23	Replenishing Congee (page 166) Go Ji Eggs (page 171) Steamed vegetables		Calamondin Roast Chicken (page 200) Yi Ren Rice (page 180) Steamed vegetables		Carp and Tofu Soup (page 211)
Day 24	Millet Congee (page 168) Green Tea Eggs (page 172) Steamed vegetables		Sautéed Ginger Chicken (page 199) Yi Ren Rice (page 180) Steamed vegetables		Pork Trotter's & Peanut Soup (page 213)
Day 25	Cornmeal Congee (page 169) Tofu Skin and Cabbage (page 175)		Rare steak Yi Ren Rice (page 180) Steamed vegetables		Dang Gui Chicken Soup (page 200)
Day 26	Quinoa Congee (page 170)		Calamondin Roast Chicken (page 200) Yi Ren Rice (page 180) Steamed vegetables		Pork Trotter's & Peanut Soup (page 213)
Day 27	Oatmeal Congee (page 168) Beijing Eggs (page 172) Sautéed greens		Sautéed Ginger Chicken (page 199) Yi Ren Rice (page 180) Steamed vegetables		Carp and Green Papaya Soup (page 212)
Day 28	Buckwheat Pilaf (page 173)		Sautéed Ginger Chicken (page 199) Yi Ren Rice (page 180) Steamed vegetables		Pork Trotter's & Peanut Soup (page 213)

Pescatarian Meal Plan

The postpartum month and months of breastfeeding are the most challenging times to forgo animal products, as they provide dense nutrition that is easy to assimilate. The less animal products you eat during the postpartum month, the more you will want to incorporate herbal formulas from a TCM herbalist, food herbs or superfoods, and dense grounding foods such as root vegetables and legumes. Nuts fall into this category but are more difficult to digest so must be taken in limited amounts. Consider adding eggs, fish, and bone broth during this time.

Stage 1 - Week 1

Treatment Principle: Detoxify the body and discharge lochia.

The focus of the first week is to gently discharge from the body the lochia and any residual contents from the womb. Water retention needs to be efficiently cleared as well. However, the body is also at its weakest, so extra care must be taken to conserve Qi and Blood.

Stage 2 - Week 2

Treatment Principle: Contract the internal organs, uterus, and pelvic cavity.

After much of the excesses have been discharged from the body, the focus of the second week is to contract everything back to its normal size.

Stage 3 - Weeks 3-4 (&5)

Treatment Principle: Nourish, supplement, and renew strength.

After two weeks the body has been cleared of toxins enough to focus primarily on tonifying. Repeat the recipes as necessary for the fifth week.

Table 11.9. Sample Pescatarian Meal Plan Week 1

	Breakfast	Tea	Lunch	Tea	Dinner
Day 1	Water Reducing Congee (page 165) Go Ji Eggs (page 171) Steamed carrots Placenta capsules	Red Date Tea (page 157) Postpartum Tea (page 158) Herbal tea from TCM herbalist	African Peanut Soup (page 216) Placenta capsules	Red Date Tea (page 157) Postpartum Tea (page 158) Herbal tea from TCM herbalist	Fish and Carrot Soup (page 210) Red Adzuki Bean Tea (page 159) Placenta capsules
Day 2	Cereal Milk (page 167) Beijing Eggs (page 172) Sautéed greens Placenta capsules		Adzuki Bean Stew (page 217) Placenta capsules		Fish and Carrot Soup (page 210) Placenta capsules
Day 3	Water Reducing Congee (page 165) Go Ji Eggs (page 171) Steamed beets Placenta capsules		Seitan Noodle Bowl (page 201) Sweet Adzuki Bean Soup (page 178) Placenta capsules		Coconut Fish Soup (page 210) Placenta capsules
Day 4	Water Reducing Congee (page 165) Green Tea Eggs (page 172) Sautéed eggplant Placenta capsules		Tempeh Tikka Masala (page 202) Yi Ren Rice (page 180)		Carp and Tofu Soup (page 211) Red Adzuki Bean Tea (page 159) Placenta capsules
Day 5	Cereal Milk (page 167) Beijing Eggs (page 172) Sautéed greens Placenta capsules		Adzuki Bean Stew (page 217)		Coconut Fish Soup (page 210) Red Adzuki Bean Tea (page 159) Placenta capsules
Day 6	Water Reducing Congee (page 165) Go Ji Eggs (page 171) Steamed carrots Placenta capsules		African Peanut Soup (page 216)		Fish and Carrot Soup (page 210) Red Adzuki Bean Tea (page 159) Placenta capsules
Day 7	Cereal Milk (page 167) Beijing Eggs (page 172) Sautéed greens Placenta capsules		Palak Tempeh (page 203)		Carp and Green Papaya Soup (page 212) Red Adzuki Bean Tea (page 159)Placenta capsules

Table 11.10. Sample Pescatarian Meal Plan Week 2

	Breakfast	Tea	Lunch	Tea	Dinner
Day 8	Cornmeal Congee (page 169) Go Ji Eggs (page 171) Steamed vegetables Placenta capsules	Postpartum Tea (page 158) Red Adzuki Bean Tea (page 159) Herbal tea from TCM herbalist	African Peanut Soup (page 216)	Postpartum Tea (page 158) Milk Kefir (page 222) Herbal tea from TCM herbalist	Fish and Carrot Soup (page 210) Red Adzuki Bean Tea (page 159) Placenta capsules
Day 9	Water Reducing Congee (page 165) Green Tea Eggs (page 172) Sautéed eggplant Placenta capsules		Adzuki Bean Stew (page 217)		Fish and Carrot Soup (page 210) Placenta capsules
Day 10	Cornmeal Congee (page 169) Go Ji Eggs (page 171) Steamed vegetables Placenta capsules		Seitan Noodle Bowl (page 201) Sweet Adzuki Bean Soup (page 178)		Coconut Fish Soup (page 210) Placenta capsules
Day 11	Cereal Milk (page 167) Beijing Eggs (page 172) Sautéed greens Placenta capsules		Tempeh Tikka Masala (page 202) Yi Ren Rice (page 180)		Carp and Tofu Soup (page 211) Red Adzuki Bean Tea (page 159) Placenta capsules
Day 12	Water Reducing Congee (page 165) Green Tea Eggs (page 172) Sautéed eggplant Placenta capsules		Adzuki Bean Stew (page 217)		Coconut Fish Soup (page 210) Red Adzuki Bean Tea (page 159) Placenta capsules
Day 13	Cereal Milk (page 167) Beijing Eggs (page 172) Sautéed greens Placenta capsules		African Peanut Soup (page 216)		Fish and Carrot Soup (page 210) Red Adzuki Bean Tea (page 159) Placenta capsules
Day 14	Water Reducing Congee (page 165) Go Ji Eggs (page 171) Sautéed eggplant Placenta capsules		Palak Tempeh (page 203)		Carp and Green Papaya Soup (page 212) Red Adzuki Bean Tea (page 159) Placenta capsules

Table 11.11. Sample Pescatarian Meal Plan Weeks 3-4 (&5)

	Breakfast	Tea	Lunch	Tea	Dinner
Day 15/22	Replenishing Congee (page 166) Go Ji Eggs (page 171) Steamed vegetables	Milk Kefir (page 222) Date and White Cloud Tea (page 160) Herbal tea from TCM herbalist	Lentil Barley Stew (page 219)	Date and White Cloud Tea (page 160) Red Adzuki Bean Tea (page 159) Herbal tea from TCM herbalist	Fish and Carrot Soup (page 210) Placenta capsules
Day 16/23	Millet Congee (page 168) Green Tea Eggs (page 172) Steamed vegetables		Polenta Lasagna (page 205)		Fish and Carrot Soup (page 210) Placenta capsules
Day 17/24	Cornmeal Congee (page 169) Tofu Skin and Cabbage (page 175)		Yi Ren Rice (page 180) Black Bean Soup (page 217) Steamed vegetables		Coconut Fish Soup (page 210) Placenta capsules
Day 18/25	Quinoa Frittata (page 173)		Pumpkin Stew (page 220)		Carp and Tofu Soup (page 211) Placenta capsules
Day 19/26	Oatmeal Congee (page 168) Beijing Eggs (page 172) Sautéed greens		Yi Ren Rice (page 180) Refried Adzuki Beans (page 178) Steamed vegetables		Coconut Fish Soup (page 210) Placenta capsules
Day 20/27	Buckwheat Pilaf (page 173)		Polenta Lasagna (page 205)		Fish and Carrot Soup (page 210) Placenta capsules
Day 21/28	Replenishing Congee (page 166) Go Ji Eggs (page 171) Steamed vegetables		Thai Curry Squash (page 204) Yi Ren Rice (page 180)		Carp and Green Papaya Soup (page 212) Placenta capsules

Vegan Meal Plan

The postpartum month and months of breastfeeding create a challenge for a vegan diet. A vegan diet tends to be more cooling and cleansing, whereas postpartum women require warming, building foods. This can be remedied with herbal formulas from a TCM herbalist, using food herbs liberally, and by eating dense grounding foods such as root vegetables and legumes. Nuts fall into this category but are more difficult to digest so must be taken in limited amounts. Consider placenta encapsulation in order to provide stronger tonification postpartum.

Stage 1 - Week 1

Treatment Principle: Detoxify the body and discharge lochia.

The focus of the first week is to gently discharge from the body the lochia and any residual contents from the womb. Water retention needs to be efficiently cleared as well. However, the body is also at its weakest, so extra care must be taken to conserve Qi and Blood.

Stage 2 - Week 2

Treatment Principle: Contract the internal organs, uterus, and pelvic cavity.

After much of the excesses have been discharged from the body, the focus of the second week is to contract everything back to its normal size.

Stage 3 - Weeks 3-4 (&5)

Treatment Principle: Nourish, supplement, and renew strength.

After two weeks the body has been cleared of toxins enough to focus primarily on tonifying. Repeat the recipes as necessary for the fifth week.

Table 11.12. Sample Vegan Meal Plan Week 1

	Breakfast	Tea	Lunch	Tea	Dinner
Day 1	Hearty Vegan Congee (page 165) Placenta capsules	Red Date Tea (page 157) Postpartum Tea (page 158) Herbal tea from TCM herbalist Chlorella tablets	African Peanut Soup (page 216) Placenta capsules	Red Date Tea (page 157) Postpartum Tea (page 158) Herbal tea from TCM herbalist Chlorella tablets	Adzuki Bean Kichari (page 179) Placenta capsules
Day 2			Adzuki Bean Stew (page 217) Placenta capsules		Lentil Barley Stew (page 219) Placenta capsules
Day 3			Seitan Noodle Bowl (page 201) Sweet Adzuki Bean Soup (page 178) Placenta capsules		Date & Squash Soup (page 219) Placenta capsules
Day 4			Tempeh Tikka Masala (page 202) Yi Ren Rice (page 180)		Adzuki Bean Stew (page 217) Placenta capsules
Day 5			Adzuki Bean Stew (page 217)		Lentil Barley Stew (page 219) Placenta capsules
Day 6			African Peanut Soup (page 216)		Black Bean Soup (page 217) Placenta capsules
Day 7			Palak Tempeh (page 203)		African Peanut Soup (page 216) Placenta capsules

Table 11.13. Sample Vegan Meal Plan Week 2

	Breakfast	Tea	Lunch	Tea	Dinner
Day 8	Hearty Vegan Congee (page 165) Placenta capsules	Postpartum Tea (page 158) Herbal tea from TCM herbalist Chlorella tablets	African Peanut Soup (page 216)	Postpartum Tea (page 158) Herbal tea from TCM herbalist Chlorella tablets	Polenta Lasagna (page 205) Placenta capsules
Day 9	Cereal Milk (page 167) Tofu Skin and Cabbage (page 175) Placenta capsules		Adzuki Bean Stew (page 217)		Thai Curry Squash (page 204) Yi Ren Rice (page 180) Placenta capsules
Day 10	Cereal Milk (page 167) Stir-Fried Tofu (page 175) Placenta capsules		Seitan Noodle Bowl (page 201) Sweet Adzuki Bean Soup (page 178)		Pumpkin Stew (page 220) Placenta capsules
Day 11	Hearty Vegan Congee (page 165) Placenta capsules		Tempeh Tikka Masala (page 202) Yi Ren Rice (page 180)		Polenta Lasagna (page 205) Placenta capsules
Day 12	Cereal Milk (page 167) Baked Tempeh (page 174) Placenta capsules		Adzuki Bean Stew (page 217)		African Peanut Soup (page 216)
Day 13	Hearty Vegan Congee (page 165) Placenta capsules		African Peanut Soup (page 216)		Pumpkin Stew (page 220) Placenta capsules
Day 14	Hearty Vegan Congee (page 165) Placenta capsules		Palak Tempeh (page 203)		Lentil Barley Stew (page 219)

Table 11.14. Sample Vegan Meal Plan Weeks 3-4 (&5)

	Breakfast	Tea	Lunch	Tea	Dinner
Day 15/22	Replenishing Congee (page 166) Stir-Fried Tofu (page 175) Steamed vegetables	Date and White Cloud Tea (page 160) Herbal tea from TCM herbalist Chlorella tablets	Lentil Barley Stew (page 219)	Longan and Beet Tea (page 159) Herbal tea from TCM herbalist	African Peanut Soup (page 216) Placenta capsules
Day 16/23	Millet Congee (page 168) Baked Tempeh (page 174) Steamed vegetables		Polenta Lasagna (page 205)		Adzuki Bean Stew (page 217) Placenta capsules
Day 17/24	Cornmeal Congee (page 169) Tofu Skin and Cabbage (page 175)		Yi Ren Rice (page 180) Black Bean Soup (page 217) Steamed vegetables		Date & Squash Soup (page 219) Placenta capsules
Day 18/25	Quinoa Frittata (page 173)		Pumpkin Stew (page 220)		Adzuki Bean Stew (page 217) Placenta capsules
Day 19/26	Oatmeal Congee (page 168) Stir-Fried Tofu (page 175) Sautéed greens		Yi Ren Rice (page 180) Refried Adzuki Beans (page 178) Steamed vegetables		Lentil Barley Stew (page 219) Placenta capsules
Day 20/27	Buckwheat Pilaf (page 173)		Polenta Lasagna (page 205)		Black Bean Soup (page 217) Placenta capsules
Day 21/28	Replenishing Congee (page 166) Stir-Fried Tofu (page 175) Steamed vegetables		Thai Curry Squash (page 204) Yi Ren Rice (page 180)		African Peanut Soup (page 216) Placenta capsules

Reference

Recipes

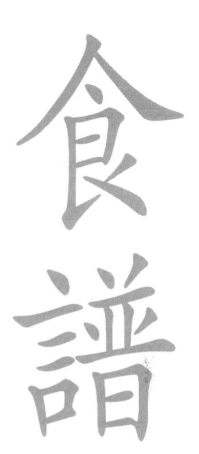

These recipes are not to entertain and impress your friends. Their purpose is to recover a woman's health quickly and completely after childbirth and while breastfeeding (or anyone after blood loss). You will love them for how they make you look and feel, and some of them for their taste. Others hopefully will grow on you.

Traditional Chinese and Taiwanese postpartum food is bland and hydrating. This approach is used for convalescent food in general. Bland, soft, moist foods are easier to digest and replenish lost fluids. Modern people are typically addicted to overstimulation and require more exciting food. I have adapted the recipes accordingly where possible. Feel free to simplify recipes and use less spices. Salt was intentionally left out of the majority of the recipes. Salt is kept to a minimum in the postpartum diet to alleviate water retention. Excess salt also injures the Blood, which is already deficient. Cook without salt and use minimal salt at the table during the Postpartum Recovery Program™.

Recipes for the Last Trimester and Delivery

One week prior to projected delivery, begin taking Red Date Tea (page 157). This protects the body in case of anesthesia. The following are recipes and formulas traditionally taken leading up to delivery to build strength and ease labor. Regular massage and acupuncture during the last month will ease discomfort and relax the body for birth. Sipping pungent teas throughout the day, such as mint, and eating spicy foods gently move Qi and Blood and help promote delivery.

Water-Clearing Tea

Comments:
During the last trimester, and particularly the last month of pregnancy, many women suffer from water retention, swelling, and joint pain. Adzuki bean (*chi xiao dou*) is an excellent food to remove excess fluids. Poria (*fu ling*) moves excess fluids, strengthens the Spleen (digestion), and calms the mind. This simple tea can be taken daily to stay comfortable. It can also be used postpartum to clear water retention. Postpartum water retention easily turns into fat and must be moved promptly.

Ingredients:
½ cup red adzuki beans (*chi xiao dou*)
3 pieces of poria (*fu ling*)
4 cups water

Preparation:
1. Soak beans overnight
2. Place ingredients in a saucepan. Bring to a boil and simmer for 45 minutes. Skim any bubbles that rise to the surface and discard.
3. Strain and serve.

How to Drink:
Drink 1 cup, 2-3 times a day as needed to keep down swelling.

Slippery Baby Congee[1]

Comments:
These mucilaginous greens ease labor, as well as promote bowel movements, ease urination, reduce swelling, and clear Heat. Choose between ma chi xian (purslane), kong xin cai (ong choy or water spinach), dong xian cai (hin choy or winter amaranth), macha, or spinach.

---

1. Adapted from Chang, Lily. "Chinese Medial Terminology." (lecture, Pacific College of Oriental Medicine, San Diego, November 2, 2007).

Ingredients:
1 cup mucilaginous greens, chopped
½ cup white jasmine rice
4 cups water

Preparation:
1. Add ingredients to crock pot or rice cooker.
2. Cook 6 hours or overnight.

How to Eat:
Have 1 bowl, three times a day. Begin 1-2 days prior to projected delivery date.

Tofu Skin Congee[2]

Comments:
This recipe eases labor as well as tonifies the Lungs and Spleen.

Ingredients:
½ cup tofu skin, chopped
½ cup white jasmine rice
raw sugar (muscovado) or other sweetener to taste (optional)
4 cups water

Preparation:
1. Add ingredients to crock pot or rice cooker.
2. Cook 6 hours or overnight.

How to Eat:
Have 1 bowl, three times a day. Begin 1-2 days prior to projected delivery date.

Tangerine & Seaweed Congee[3]

Comments:
This recipe transforms Phlegm-Damp. It can be used to promote menses as well as labor. Kelp is preferred for diet therapy as it is the strongest of the seaweeds. Any seaweed can be used in its place with slight variation of effects.

---

2. Ibid.
3. Ibid.

Ingredients:
5 inch piece kelp seaweed (*kun bu*)
½ cup white jasmine rice
1 tsp. tangerine peel (*chen pi*)
4 cups of water

Preparation:
1. Place all ingredients in a rice cooker or crock pot.
2. Cook for 6 hours or overnight.

How to Eat:
Have 1 bowl, three times a day. Begin 1-2 days prior to projected delivery date.

Honey Water[4]

Comments:
Honey water is traditionally used to give women energy during delivery. Honey not only is a sugar, providing quick energy, it is moistening and facilitates the downward process of birth.

Ingredients:
2/3 cup raw honey
1 cup water

Preparation:
1. Bring water to a boil.
2. Remove from heat and stir in honey. Allow it to cool.

How to Drink:
Begin taking as soon as water breaks. It shortens labor and reduces pain.

---

4. Shuqi Zhuang. *Postpartum Recovery Program; a Manual of Rules and Recipes for the Postpartum Woman.* (Taiwan: Guang He Chu Ban She, 2005). ISBN 9578807015

Tea Recipes

Drink only warm water or tea during the postpartum month. These teas are tasty and alleviate postpartum symptoms.

Chinese Herb Decoction

Comments:
Chinese herbal formulas are given to promote the passage of lochia, nourish the body, and promote healthy breast milk. If you use raw herbs this is the method to brew them.

Preparation:
1. Rinse herbs. Soak for 30 min.
2. Place herbs with 4-5 cups of water in non-aluminum pot. Bring to a boil, then simmer for 45 minutes.
3. Strain. Conserve decoction and herbs.
4. Return herbs to pot with 3-4 cups of water. Bring to a boil and simmer for 45 minutes.
5. Strain. Discard herbs. Combine the two decoctions.

How to Drink:
Drink 1 cup warmed decoction, 1-3 times a day.

Red Date Tea

Comments:
Red dates (*hong zao*) neutralize toxins, protect the Liver, and tonify Qi and Blood. Red Date Tea is indicated one week prior and two weeks after anesthesia (often used in childbirth).[5] Also it strengthens the body during the postpartum period. Wood ear mushroom is often added postpartum as it moves blood circulation and decongests fluids.

Ingredients (2 day's dosage):
7 large red dates (*hong zao*), split and pit removed
1 large wood ear mushroom (*hei mu er*) (optional)
3 cups water

Preparation:
1. Rinse red dates with warm water. Use a knife to cut open the fruits. Soak dates and wood ear mushroom in water for 30 minutes.
2. Put ingredients into a pot. Bring to a boil and simmer for 1 hour.

---

5. Possible side effects from anesthesia include: flatulence, hair loss, insomnia, memory loss, constipation, and other symptoms.

3. Strain decoction and serve.

How to Drink:

Drink warmed 1-2 cups a day.

Postpartum Tea[6]

Comments:

This tea removes excess water weight, moves the Blood, and hydrates the body. Dr. Shuqi Zhuang recommends using hawthorn berries (*shan zha*), lychee shells (*li zhi ke*),[7] and clerodendri (*guan yin*)[8] to equal 600g. I recommend using a smaller proportion of hawthorn berries to avoid hyperacidity in the Stomach. If you have acid reflux, omit hawthorn berries and add 1 large wood ear fungus (*hei mu er*). Rose flower (*mei gui hua*) moves stagnant energy (Liver Qi) in the body and is sometimes included in postpartum teas.

Ingredients (10 day supply):

100g (1 ½ cups) hawthorn berries (*shan zha*)

200g lychee shells (*li zhi ke*)

200g clerodendri (*guan yin*)

40g (1 cup) rose flower (*mei gui hua*)

raw sugar (muscovado), or other sweetener to taste (optional)

1 ½ gallons water

Preparation:

1. Rinse herbs and put them in a non-aluminum pot with water.

2. Place pot over high heat, cover. Bring to a boil and reduce to low heat. Simmer for1 hour.

3. Strain. Store decoction and discard herbs.

How to Drink:

Drink warm throughout the day to hydrate the body and allay postpartum symptoms.

---

6. Shuqi Zhuang. *Postpartum Recovery Program; a Manual of Rules and Recipes for the Postpartum Woman.* (Taiwan: Guang He Chu Ban She, 2005). ISBN 9578807015

7. Lychee shell (荔枝殼, lì zhī ké) is used in TCM to alleviate postpartum thirst and treat abdominal bloating. It is also used to treat smallpox rashes, metrorrhagia (irregular menstrual bleeding and spotting), leukorrhea (pathological vaginal discharge), and externally for eczema. It is cool and bitter and goes to the Heart channel. Be sure to source it from clean sources that test for pesticides as the shell is more likely to be affected. Not much is available on lychee shells' use in TCM in English. For more in Chinese see www.baike.baidu.com/view/756081.htm?fr=wordsearch

8. Clerodendri (觀音串, guān yīn chuàn) is used in the Taiwanese postpartum tradition to reduce water weight, "shrink" the lower abdomen after delivery, and alleviate thirst. It is bitter and neutral, tonifies and raises Spleen Qi, and moves Blood. It is used to treat fatigue, uterine prolapse, childhood malnutrition, edema, clear leukorrhea (pathological vaginal discharge), Wind Damp Bi (joint pain caused by Dampness), low back weakness, irregular menses, dysmenorrhea (menstrual cramps), and traumatic injuries. Not much is available on clerodendri's use in TCM in English. For more in Chinese see www.baike.baidu.com/view/1800810.htm

Red Adzuki Bean Tea

Comments:

This is the easiest way to include red adzuki beans (*chi xiao dou*) in the diet. Adzuki beans move the Blood and drain excess water from the body.

Ingredients:

1 cup red adzuki beans (*chi xiao dou*)
1 bay leaf
1-2 tsp. coriander
1 inch piece fresh ginger, chopped
raw sugar (muscovado), or other sweetener to taste (optional)
4 cups water
dash of rice wine (optional)

Preparation:

1. Soak beans 8 hours or overnight.
2. Place beans, rice wine (optional), and water in saucepan. Bring to a boil and skim off bubbles.
3. Add bay leaf, coriander, and ginger. Simmer for 1 hour or until beans are thoroughly cooked.
4. Strain tea and discard beans. Add sweetener (optional) and serve.

How to Drink:

Drink a cup of warmed Adzuki Bean Tea 1-2 times a day, with or between meals.

Longan and Beet Tea

Comments:

This tea tonifies Blood, beautifies the skin, calms anxiety, and eases sleep. It can be taken regularly anytime but is particularly helpful after blood loss or breast feeding.

Ingredients (2-3 day supply):

½ cup longan berries (*long yan rou*)
2 tbsp. beet powder
12 lotus nuts (*lian zi*)
raw sugar (muscovado), or other sweetener to taste (optional)
3 cups water

A FIX FOR SLEEPLESS NIGHTS

I had a patient who suffered from insomnia for 10 years that was getting worse as she neared menopause. She was sensitive to herbs and medications. After three nights of taking this tea she was able to sleep through the night and wake up feeling rested.

Preparation:

1. Rinse longan berries and lotus nuts and put them in a pot with water. Soak for 30 minutes.
2. Place the pot over high heat, cover. Bring to a boil and reduce to low heat. Simmer for 45 minutes.
3. The herbs can either be strained or eaten with the tea as preferred. Stir in beet powder and sweetener if desired.

How to Drink:
Drink warm 1-2 times a day to hydrate the body and boost the Blood.

Date and White Cloud Tea

Comments:
This tea nourishes Yin and body fluids, beautifies the skin, calms anxiety, and hydrates the body. It is popular as a tea or dessert to plump up the skin and prevent wrinkles and can be taken regularly anytime. It is particularly helpful after blood loss or during breast feeding. The proportion of ingredients can be increased to the amount of water to make a dessert soup. Papaya is another traditional ingredient and can be added during the last 5-10 minutes of simmering.

Ingredients (2-3 day supply):
1 piece white cloud mushroom (*bai mu er*)
4 large red dates (*hong zao*), split and pits removed
1 tbsp. go ji berries (*go qi zi*)
6 lotus nuts (*lian zi*)
1 tbsp. lily bulbs (*bai he*) (optional)
raw sugar (muscovado), or other sweetener to taste (optional)
3 cups water

Preparation:

1. Rinse herbs and put them in a pot with water. Soak for 45 min.
2. Remove the hard base from the white cloud mushroom and discard. Remove pits from dates. Add sugar if desired.
3. Place the pot over high heat, cover. Bring to a boil and reduce to low heat. Simmer for 1 hour.
4. The herbs can either be strained or eaten with the tea as preferred.

How to Drink:
Drink warm 1-2 times a day to hydrate the body.

Hawthorn Berry Tea

Comments:
Hawthorn berry (*shan zha*) moves the Blood (aids circulation), dissolves Food stagnation (is a digestive, particularly for protein), and resolves abdominal pain. This tea is particularly helpful if you are passing clots in your lochia (or menses). However, hawthorn berries are very sour and can aggravate hyperacidity in the stomach. Avoid if you suffer from acid reflux.

Ingredients (3 day's dosage):
100g (1 ½ cups) hawthorn berry (*shan zha*)
4 ½ cups water
raw sugar (muscovado), or other sweetener to taste (optional)

Preparation:
1. Rinse hawthorn berries. Place hawthorn berries and water in a non-aluminum pot. Soak for 30 minutes.
2. Place over high heat, covered, and bring to a boil. Reduce to low heat and simmer for 45 minutes.
3. Strain decoction. If desired, add sweetener to taste. Mix well and turn off heat. It is ready to serve.

How to Drink:
The daily dosage is about 1 cup. Take small amounts several times throughout the day for three days in a row. This will dissolve congealed blood (clots) and alleviate abdominal pain.

Roasted Mai Ya Tea (Sprouted Barley Tea)

Comments:
Roasted sprouted barley stops lactation, eases breast distention, and dissolves Food stagnation.

Ingredients (3 day's dosage):
180g sprouted barley (*mai ya*, malt)
8 cups of water
brown sugar or other sweetener (optional)

Preparation:
1. If sprouted barley is not already toasted, dry fry it in a frying pan until slightly browned but not burnt.
2. Place sprouted barley and 8 cups of water in a non-aluminum pot and bring to a boil over high heat. Cover. Lower to low heat and simmer for 1 hour.
3. Strain decoction into an uncovered pot. Bring to a boil over high heat and reduce to about 6 cups. Add brown sugar and mix thoroughly. Turn off heat and serve.

How to Drink:
Divide into six doses; about 1 cup each. For three consecutive days, take two doses per day: the first after breakfast, the second after dinner.

Breakfast Recipes

Congee Recipes

Liver Congee #1 (Traditional Taiwanese Recovery Recipe)[9]

Comments:

This is a traditional recipe Dr. Shuqi Zhuang recommends for the first three days after a C-section delivery. Pork liver is one of the strongest foods to nourish Blood and Yin. Chinese yam nourishes Qi, Yin, and body fluids. Chinese yam, foxnuts, and lotus seeds astringe fluids assisting the body to recover from fluid loss. Excessive blood loss generates tremendous thirst as the body attempts to recover fluids. Without astringents, water intake will exit quickly via urination and the body is constantly trying to catch up. Coix seed tonifies Qi and also clear Heat, Dampness, and Toxins. Even though it is highly effective, unmodified, this recipe is unpalatable to most Westerners (see next recipe).

Ingredients:

200g (7 oz) organic pork liver, chopped
200g (7 oz) fresh Chinese yam (*shan yao*), peeled and chopped
500g (17 oz) coix seed (*yi yi ren*)
20g (0.7 oz) poria (*fu ling*)
50g (1.7 oz) lotus nuts (*lian zi*)
15g (0.5) foxnuts (*qian shi*)
10 gingko nuts (*bai guo*), shelled
500cc (2 cups) rice wine or Zuo Yue Zi water

Preparation:

1. Rinse dry ingredients.
2. Add all ingredients to a rice cooker and set to "porridge." Alternately, place ingredients in a crock pot or slow cooker set to low.
3. Cook 6 hours or overnight.

How to Eat:

Eat 1 bowl for breakfast and lunch for three days after a C-section.

---

9. Adapted from Shuqi Zhuang. *Postpartum Recovery Program; a Manual of Rules and Recipes for the Postpartum Woman.* (Taiwan: Guang He Chu Ban She, 2005). ISBN 9578807015

Liver Congee #2 (Canja de Figado)[10]

Comments:

This congee is a superb Blood-builder and a modification of the traditional recipe. It is eaten during the first week postpartum. I replaced pork liver with chicken liver as it is more palatable, even though pork liver is better therapeutically. Chicken livers have a hot thermal temperature, whereas pork livers are neutral and nourish Yin as well as Blood. I added tomato as it moves Qi and Blood and improves the taste. Rice and herbs also harmonize the flavor and increase digestibility. Note: foxnuts (*qian shi*) have a strong ability to make an entire recipe bland. Omit if this is a problem.

Ingredients:

½ lb. organic chicken liver
1 cup of white jasmine rice
1 large tomato, skin and seeds removed, chopped
2 inch piece fresh Chinese yam (*shan yao*), peeled and chopped, or 2 pieces dried
6 lotus nuts (*lian zi*)
¼ cup coix seed (*yi yi ren*)
2 pieces poria (*fu ling*)
1 tbsp. foxnuts (*qian shi*)
6 gingko nuts (*bai guo*), shelled
1 small onion, chopped
1 clove of garlic
1 bunch parsley, chopped
1 bunch marjoram, chopped (optional)
½ inch fresh ginger, chopped
1 lime or lemon
olive oil to coat pan
dash of rice wine (or dry sherry)
4 cups soup stock or water

Preparation:

1. Rinse lotus nuts, poria, fox nuts, gingko nuts, and coix seed and soak for 30 minutes.
2. Rinse rice in a colander.
3. Add oil to a saucepan and place over high heat. Add ginger and garlic and sauté until they begin to brown. Add rice and sauté for 1 minute.
4. Add tomato, parsley, marjoram, Chinese herbs, Chinese yam, and stock. Bring to a boil and simmer for 1 hour.

---

10. Adapted from Deborah. (2013). *Sopa de Fígado de Frango*. Retrieved from www.delicias1001.com.br/2013/03/sopa-de-figado-de-frango.html

5. Meanwhile, rinse livers and place in a bowl. Cover with lime juice and allow to sit for 30 minutes. Strain livers.
6. Add oil to frying pan and place over high heat. Add onions and sauté until browned. Add livers and sauté until browned. Lower heat and cook until partially cooked but still soft. Remove from heat and crumble into tiny pieces. Add to rice congee and mix.

How to Eat:
Eat a bowl for breakfast or whenever you desire to quickly recover from blood and fluid loss.

Canja de Galinha[11]

Comments:
This congee tonifies Qi and Blood and supports lactation. It is eaten during the third and fourth weeks postpartum.

Ingredients:
¾ cup white rice
4 organic chicken thighs (or 1 breast)
½ cup frozen peas
1 tsp. thyme, tarragon
1 small onion, chopped
1 bunch parsley, chopped
½ inch fresh ginger, chopped
olive oil
5 cups water or soup stock

Preparation:
1. Rinse rice in a colander.
2. Add oil to a saucepan and place over medium-high heat.
3. Add onions and ginger and sauté until they begin to brown. Add chicken and sauté until it gets some color. Add rice and sauté for 1 minute.
4. Add water or soup stock, parsley, thyme, tarragon, and peas. Bring to a boil and simmer for 1 hour. Using a fork, pull the meat from the bones and shred. Discard the bones. Put the meat back in the congee and stir.

How to Eat:
Eat a bowl for breakfast or whenever you desire.

---

11. Based on my mom, Dr. Judith Andrews', recipe.

Hearty Vegan Congee

Comments:

This congee has added protein and warmth to nourish women postpartum. Adzuki beans clear water retention, move lochia, and promote lactation. Coix seed clears water retention and inflammation.

Ingredients:

¼ cup white sweet (glutinous) rice
¼ cup short grain brown rice
¼ cup red adzuki beans (*chi xiao dou*)
¼ cup coix seed (*yi yi ren*)
½ cup tofu skin, chopped (or firm tofu)
½ cup sweet potato, chopped
2 inch piece fresh Chinese yam (*shan yao*), peeled and chopped, or 2 pieces dried
¼ cup walnuts (*hu tao ren*)
¼ cup go ji berries (*go qi zi*)
¼ cup black sesame seeds (*hei zhi ma*)
6 lotus nuts (*lian zi*)
2 stalks of celery, chopped
dash of rice wine (or sherry)
3 slices of fresh ginger
6 cups water

Preparation:

1. Rinse rice, beans, and coix seed in a colander and soak for 6-8 hours. Strain.
2. Add all ingredients to a rice cooker or crock pot. If using a rice cooker set to "porridge." If using a crock pot, set on low and leave overnight.

How to Eat:

Eat a bowl for breakfast or whenever you desire.

Water Reducing Congee

Comments:

This recipe combines several key postpartum ingredients: red adzuki beans, coix seed, sweet rice, and ginger. It clears water retention, promotes lactation, moves Blood, gently detoxifies, and is excellent to reduce excess weight.

Ingredients:

1/3 cup red adzuki beans (*chi xiao dou*)
¼ cup coix seed (*yi yi ren*)
¼ cup white sweet (glutinous) rice

¼ cup of white jasmine rice

3 slices of fresh ginger

6 longan berries (*long yan rou*)

1 piece of tangerine peel (*chen pi*) (optional)

5 cups of water

raw sugar (muscovado), or other sweetener to taste (optional)

Preparation:
1. Sauté ginger in saucepan over high heat until browned.
2. Place ingredients in crock pot or rice cooker and cook overnight.

How to Eat:
Eat 1 bowl first thing in the morning with a protein and vegetable dish.

Replenishing Congee

Comments:
Sweet rice is a stronger Qi and Blood tonic. However it is a little heavy and best mixed with white rice such as jasmine rice. Chinese yam (*shan yao*), go ji berries (*go qi zi*), longan berries (*long yan rou*), and black sesame seeds (*hei zhi ma*) nourish Blood, Yin, and body fluids. Choose between astragalus (*huang qi*) and codonopsis root (*dang shen*) to strengthen Qi.

Ingredients:
¼ cup jasmine rice

¼ cup white sweet (glutinous) rice

2 inch piece fresh Chinese yam (*shan yao*), peeled and chopped, or 2 pieces dried

¼ cup coix seed (*yi yi ren*)

3 pieces astragalus (*huang qi*) or 2 pieces codonopsis root (*dang shen*) from a TCM herbalist

6 longan berries (*long yan rou*)

1 heaping tbsp. go ji berries (*go qi zi*)

1 tbsp. black sesame seed (*hei zhi ma*)

5 cups water

raw sugar (muscovado), or other sweetener to taste (optional)

Preparation:
1. Rinse dry ingredients. Add all ingredients to a rice cooker and set to "porridge." Alternately, place ingredients in a crock pot or slow cooker set to low.
2. Cook 6 hours or overnight.

How to Eat:
Eat 1 bowl for breakfast with a protein and vegetable dish.

Simple Sweet Rice Congee

Comments:
The addition of longan berries (*long yan rou*) strengthens the Qi and Blood, calms anxiety, beautifies the skin, and treats insomnia. Sweet rice has a stronger action to tonify Qi and Blood. It is important to eat sweet rice in moderation as it can be difficult to digest and can cause flatulence and indigestion when eaten in excess.

Ingredients:
¼ cup white sweet (glutinous) rice
¼ cup white jasmine rice
6 longan berries (*long yan rou*)
4 cups water
dash of rice wine or dry sherry
raw sugar (muscovado) to taste (optional)

Preparation:
1. Soak sweet rice for 8 hours or overnight.
2. Soak herbs for 30 min.
3. Put all ingredients into rice cooker (set on porridge) or crock pot. Cook for 8 hours. On the stovetop, put ingredients into pot. Bring to a boil over high heat, then reduce heat and simmer for 8 hours.
4. Add sweetener if desired and serve.

How to Eat:
Eat 1 bowl for breakfast with a protein and vegetable dish.

Cereal Milk

Comments:
Cereal milk is traditional breakfast in many Asian cultures. It provides easily assimilated nutrients similar to congee and is ideal for those with limited appetite in the morning. This particular mix nourishes Blood and Jing and supports lactation.

Ingredients:
1 tbsp. cup coix seed (*yi yi ren*)
2 tbsp. black sesame seeds (*hei zhi ma*)
1 tbsp. oats
1 tbsp. brown rice
1 tbsp. white sweet (glutinous) rice
raw sugar (muscovado) to taste (optional)
2 cups of water

Preparation:

1. Grind dry ingredients in a blender or food processor to a fine powder and store.
2. Bring water to a boil in a saucepan. Slowly add powder while whisking continuously to prevent clumps. Lower heat to a simmer and continues to whisk as needed for 10 minutes until mixture is fully cooked.

How to Eat:

Drink warm first thing in the morning.

Oatmeal Congee

Comments:

This congee is ideal for women who require added protein and warmth. Oats are warming and high in protein. Poria (*fu ling*) tonifies Qi and clears excess water and Dampness. Hemp seeds (*huo ma ren*) and mulberries (*sang shen*) nourish Yin and Blood and promote regular bowel movement.

Ingredients:

½ cup Steel Cut (Irish) or Scottish (finer ground) oats
12g poria (fu ling)
1 heaping tbsp. hemp seeds (*huo ma ren*)
1 heaping tbsp. dried mulberries (*sang shen*) (if unavailable add ¼ cup strawberries, blackberries, etc.)
pinch of cinnamon or nutmeg
5 cups water
raw sugar (muscovado) to taste (optional)

Preparation:

1. Rinse dry ingredients.
2. Add all ingredients to a rice cooker and set to "porridge." Alternately, place ingredients in a crock pot or slow cooker set to low.
3. Cook 6 hours or overnight.

How to Eat:

Eat 1 bowl for breakfast with a protein and vegetable dish.

Millet Congee

Comments:

This congee is ideal for women who feel dry, dehydrated, and are running hot. Millet is cooling and nourishes Yin and body fluids. Coix seed (*yi yi ren*) tonify Qi and clear Dampness,

Heat, and toxins. Lotus nuts (*lian zi*) astringe fluids and tonify Qi, while longan berries (*long yan rou*) tonify Qi and Blood and calm the Shen.

Ingredients:
¼ cup jasmine rice
¼ cup millet
¼ cup coix seed (*yi yi ren*)
6 lotus nuts (*lian zi*)
6 longan berries (*long yan rou*)
5 cups water
raw sugar (muscovado) to taste (optional)

Preparation:
1. Rinse dry ingredients.
2. Add all ingredients to a rice cooker and set to "porridge." Alternately, place ingredients in a crock pot or slow cooker set to low.
3. Cook 6 hours or overnight.

How to Eat:
Eat 1 bowl for breakfast with a protein and vegetable dish.

Cornmeal Congee

Comments:
This congee helps drain water weight while building Qi and Blood. Whole grain cornmeal has a neutral temperature, strengthens the Kidneys, and regulates digestion. The addition of figs and hemp seeds (*huo ma ren*) nourish Blood and promote bowel regularity. Red dates (*hong zao*) tonify Qi and Blood and protect the Liver. Poria (*fu ling*) tonifies Qi and clears excess water and Dampness.

Ingredients:
½ cup whole grain cornmeal
4 red dates (*hong zao*), split and pitted
4 dried figs, chopped
3 pieces of poria (*fu ling*)
1 heaping tbsp. hemp seeds (*huo ma ren*)
5 cups water
raw sugar (muscovado) to taste (optional)

Preparation:
1. Rinse dry ingredients.

2. Add all ingredients to a rice cooker and set to "porridge." Alternately, place ingredients in a crock pot or slow cooker set to low.
3. Cook 6 hours or overnight.

How to Eat:
Eat 1 bowl for breakfast with a protein and vegetable dish.

Quinoa Congee

Comments:
This congee is ideal for women who require added protein and warmth. Quinoa is warming, tonifies Qi and Yang, and is high in protein. Poria (*fu ling*) tonifies Qi and clears excess water and Dampness. Go ji berries (*go qi zi*) nourish Blood and Yin. Chia seeds create a creamier consistency, promote bowel regularity, and nourish Yin.

Ingredients:
½ cup quinoa
3 pieces of poria (*fu ling*)
1 heaping tbsp. go ji berries (*go qi zi*)
1 heaping tbsp. chia seeds
5 cups water
raw sugar (muscovado) to taste (optional)

Preparation:
1. Rinse dry ingredients.
2. Add all ingredients to a rice cooker and set to "porridge." Alternately, place ingredients in a crock pot or slow cooker set to low.
3. Cook 6 hours or overnight.

How to Eat:
Eat 1 bowl for breakfast with a protein and vegetable dish.

Egg Recipes

Eggs should be eaten the entire month postpartum as they nourish Yin and Blood, promote lactation, and help recover the body after illness.

Pickled Eggs[12]

Comments:

This is a traditional Chinese postpartum recipe. The addition of vinegar makes the eggs more digestible, and helps move the circulation.

Ingredients (5 day's dosage):

10 raw eggs
1 bottle of rice or black rice vinegar
1 lb. of fresh ginger, chopped
raw sugar (muscovado) to taste (optional)

Preparation:

1. Thirty days prior to projected delivery, put all ingredients in a pot (except sugar) and bring to a boil. Simmer for 15 min.
2. Remove from heat and mix in sugar.
3. Cool and refrigerate for 30 days.

How to Eat:

After delivery, eat 2 eggs a day for 5 days.

Go Ji Eggs[13]

Comments:

This recipe nourishes Qi, Blood, and Yin.

Ingredients:

2 eggs
1 tbsp. go ji berries (*go qi zi*)
1 tsp. grated fresh ginger
black sesame oil to coat pan

Preparation:

1. Scramble eggs in a bowl. Add go ji berries.
2. Coat frying pan with black sesame oil and place over medium high heat.
3. Add ginger and sauté until ginger is browned and fragrant, but not blackened.
4. Lower heat to medium low. Add egg mixture. Sauté until cooked through. Serve.

How to Eat:

Eat with your choice of congee and fruit or vegetable.

---

12. Shaoting Jing. "TCM Gynecology." (lecture, Yo San University, Los Angeles, May 15, 2003).
13. Adapted from a dish served at Jing Mommy meal service (www.JingMommy.com).

Green Tea Eggs[14]

Comments:
This recipe renders the eggs more digestible.

Ingredients:
4 hardboiled eggs
1 tbsp. green tea
1 tbsp. hawthorn berry (*shan zha*)
1 tsp. tangerine peel (*chen pi*)
soy sauce to taste
 2 cups of water

Preparation:
1. Make little cracks in the egg shells but do not remove the shells.
2. Place ingredients in a sauce pan and bring to a boil.
3. Simmer for 30 minutes.
4. Remove eggs and discard tea.

How to Eat:
Eat eggs as a snack.

Beijing Eggs with Tomato

Comments:
Tomato and chili counter the cloying, congesting nature of the eggs.

Ingredients:
2 eggs
2 tomatoes, diced
black sesame oil to coat pan
½ tsp. red chili bean paste

Preparation:
1. Scramble eggs in a bowl.
2. Add sesame oil to frying pan and place over medium-high heat.
3. Add eggs and sauté until slightly undercooked. Remove and put into bowl.
4. Add tomatoes and red chili bean paste to frying pan. Reduce to low and cover.
5. Cook until tomatoes are thoroughly cooked.
6. Add eggs back into pan and stir.

---

14. Adapted from Maoshing Ni. (lecture, Yo San University, Los Angeles, May 5, 2000).

How to Eat:
Eat eggs for breakfast or as a snack.

Buckwheat Pilaf [15]

Comments:
Buckwheat has a neutral temperature, dries Dampness, and is high in protein. This recipe is a complete meal. Omit eggs if vegan.

Ingredients:
½ cup roasted buckwheat (kasha)
1 medium red potato, scrubbed and cubed
½ cup mushrooms, chopped in small pieces
1 tbsp. go ji berries (*go qi zi*)
½ medium onion, chopped
½ inch fresh ginger, finely chopped
1 clove garlic, minced
1 small bunch parsley, chopped
1 cup boiling water
2 eggs, cooked to your liking
black sesame oil to coat pan

Preparation:
1. Coat large frying pan with oil and place over medium-high heat. Add onions, ginger, and garlic. Sauté until they begin to brown. Then add mushrooms and sauté until they begin to brown as well.
2. Lower heat to medium and add potatoes. Cook for 2 minutes covered.
3. Add buckwheat and boiling water. Turn to low. Cover and simmer for 15 minutes.
4. Meanwhile, coat a small frying pan with oil and place over medium heat. Add eggs and fry until done to your taste.
5. Add parsley to buckwheat mixture.
6. Place a serving of the buckwheat mixture on a plate and top with a serving of eggs.

How to Eat:
Complete meal.

Quinoa Frittata

Comments:
Quinoa and cheese add extra protein to this recipe.

---

15. Modified from "Kasha Breakfast Pilaf" (Delicious Living, February 2014), 40.

Ingredients:
4 eggs
½ cup cooked quinoa
¼ cup parmesan cheese
1 cup zucchini, carrots, celery, onions, and mushrooms
pinch of thyme, tarragon, and basil
pepper to taste
black sesame oil to coat griddle

Preparation:
1. Process vegetables in food processor.
2. Beat eggs and add pepper.
3. Mix ingredients. Add herbs and parmesan cheese.
4. Add black sesame oil to skillet over med-high heat. Add egg mixture.
5. Allow to cook for a few minutes, then flip. Allow to cook for a few more minutes.
6. Remove from skillet and serve.

How to Eat:
Complete meal.

Vegan Recipes

Baked Tempeh[16]

Comments:
Tempeh is an excellent source of protein for those avoiding or limiting animal products. This recipe warms up tempeh's cooling nature.

Ingredients:
1 tempeh cake (8 ounces), chop or leave whole as desired
2 tbsp. tamari or shoyu soy sauce
1 tbsp. rice wine or dry sherry
½ inch fresh ginger, grated
black sesame oil to coat pan

Preparation:
1. Marinate tempeh in other ingredients for 1 hour or overnight.
2. Preheat oven to 375° F.
3. Coat baking pan with black sesame oil and place tempeh and marinade in the pan.

---

16. Adapted from Crescent Dragonwagon. (2005). *Basic Oven-Baked Marinated Tempeh.* Retrieved from www.epicurious.com/recipes/food/views/Basic-Oven-Baked-Marinated-Tempeh-231049#ixzz2VqnvsGJZ

4. Bake 15 minutes. Flip tempeh and bake additional 15 minutes.
5. Remove from oven and serve.

How to Eat:
Eat with your choice of congee and fruit or vegetable.

Stir-Fried Tofu

Comments:
Nourishes and moves Qi and Blood.

Ingredients:
½ of firm tofu cut into cubes
1 clove garlic, minced
¼ cup shitake mushrooms, finely chopped
½ carrot, finely chopped
3 slices of fresh ginger
black sesame oil to coat pan
dash of rice wine

Preparation:
1. Add black sesame oil to sauce pan and bring over medium-high heat. Add ginger and garlic and sauté until they begin to brown.
2. Add tofu and sear.
3. Lower heat and add vegetables and rice wine. Cook for 15 minutes.

How to Eat:
Use to replace a meat dish.

Tofu Skin and Cabbage

Comments:
Nourishes and moves Qi and Blood.

Ingredients:
½ cup oyster mushrooms, chopped length-wise
½ cup tofu (bean curd) skins, chopped (if unavailable substitute firm tofu or seitan)
½ cup cabbage, chopped
¼ cup go ji berries (go qi zi)
½ onion, chopped
1 clove garlic, minced
½ inch fresh ginger, grated
tamari or soy sauce to taste

1 tbsp. black bean sauce
black sesame oil to coat pan
dash of rice wine

Preparation:
1. Put sesame oil in frying pan over med-high heat. Add ginger, garlic, and onions. Sauté until browned.
2. Add rest of the ingredients. Reduce to low heat. Stir and cover. Cook for 10-20min.
3. Remove from heat and serve.

How to Eat:
Eat with congee.

Lunch Recipes

Adzuki Bean Recipes

Adzuki beans should be eaten daily for the first 2 weeks postpartum. They can be decocted as a tea and taken with meals, eaten as regular beans, as a dessert, or added to soups and congee. When cooking beans the following tips will optimize their digestibility:

1. Soak beans 8 hours or overnight, then strain before cooking. This begins the sprouting process and increases digestibility.
2. Bring to a boil and simmer uncovered for 20 minutes, skimming bubbles off the surface.
3. Add bay leaf or seaweed while cooking.
4. At the end of cooking, sauté seasoning (such as onions, garlic, and herbs and spices) in oil and combine with cooked beans.

Red Adzuki Bean Tea

Comments:
This is the easiest way to include red adzuki beans (*chi xiao dou*) in the diet. Adzuki beans move the Blood and drain excess water from the body.

Ingredients:
1 cup red adzuki beans (*chi xiao dou*)
1 bay leaf
1-2 tsp. coriander
1 inch piece fresh ginger, chopped
raw sugar (muscovado), or other sweetener to taste (optional)
4 cups water
dash of rice wine (optional)

Preparation:
1. Soak beans 8 hours or overnight.
2. Place beans, rice wine (optional), and water in saucepan. Bring to a boil and skim off bubbles.
3. Add bay leaf, coriander, and ginger. Simmer for 1 hour or until beans are thoroughly cooked.
4. Strain tea and discard beans. Add sweetener (optional) and serve.

How to Drink:
Drink a cup of warmed Adzuki Bean Tea 1-2 times a day, with or between meals.

Sweet Adzuki Bean Soup

Comments:
This is the same recipe as Adzuki Bean Tea, but with less water. It is common in Asian cooking to eat adzuki beans (*chi xiao dou*) in desserts or as sweet soup.

Ingredients:
1 cup red adzuki beans (*chi xiao dou*)
2 cups water
1 bay leaf
1 tsp. coriander
1 inch fresh ginger, chopped
raw sugar (muscovado), or other sweetener to taste
dash of rice wine (optional)

Procedure:
1. Soak beans 8 hours or overnight.
2. Place beans and water in saucepan. Bring to a boil and skim off bubbles.
3. Add bay leaf, coriander, and ginger. Add dash of rice wine (optional). Simmer for 1 hour or until beans are thoroughly cooked.
4. Add sweetener (optional) and serve.

How to Eat:
Eat a small bowl as a dessert or snack.

Refried Adzuki Beans

Ingredients:
1 cup red adzuki beans (*chi xiao dou*)
3 cups of water
1 bay leaf
1 tsp. each cumin and thyme
3 sundried tomatoes, sliced
1 inch fresh ginger, chopped
1 small onion, finely chopped
1 bunch parsley, chopped
dash of rice wine (optional)
cooking oil to coat pan

Preparation:
1. Soak beans 8 hours or overnight.
2. Place beans, rice wine (optional), and water in saucepan. Bring to a boil and skim off bubbles.

3. Add bay leaf, cumin, and thyme. Simmer for 1 hour or until beans are thoroughly cooked.
4. In a small saucepan add oil and place over medium-high heat. Add onion and ginger. Sauté until browned. Add sun dried tomatoes and stir.
5. Add some of the cooked beans to the sautéed onion and ginger and stir. Add parsley.
6. Add sautéed beans back in the pot of boiled beans. Serve warm.

How to Eat:

Savory beans can be eaten with Yi Ren Rice.

Adzuki Bean Kichari

Comments:

This is an easy to digest, complete meal.

Ingredients:

½ cup red adzuki beans (*chi xiao dou*)
½ cup white basmati rice
½ cup sweet potato or yam, chopped
½ cup celery, chopped
1tbsp. go ji berries (*go qi zi*)
1 bay leaf
1 tsp. each cumin and thyme
1 inch piece fresh ginger, chopped
1 small onion, finely chopped
1 bunch parsley, chopped
6 cups of water
dash of rice wine (optional)
cooking oil to coat pan

Preparation:

1. Soak beans 8 hours or overnight. If using brown rice, soak it as well. Strain.
2. Coat a small saucepan with oil and place over high heat. Add onions and ginger and sauté until browned. Add cumin and thyme.
3. Add rice, beans, and vegetables. Sauté.
4. Place all ingredients in a rice cooker or crockpot and cook for 6 hours. Serve warm.

How to Eat:

Eat 1 bowl as a complete meal.

Rice Recipes

Eat white rice during the first 2 weeks as it is easier to digest. In later stages, brown rice can be used, but should be soaked and sprouted before cooking to increase digestibility.

Yi Ren Rice

Comments:
This is a traditional postpartum recipe in both Chinese and Taiwanese traditions. Coix seed has several functions that make it an ideal food postpartum. It strengthens the Spleen, leeches out Dampness (reduces edema), expels Wind-Damp (joint pain), and clears Damp-Heat (balances the tonifying diet). It also has a slightly cool temperature. Raw coix seed (*yi yi ren*) drains edema and Heat. Roasted coix seed (*yi yi ren*) tonifies the Spleen.

> **HEALING GRAIN**
>
> Rice enjoys near sacred status in Chinese culture. I can relate to this as rice is also the staple grain in my mom's native Brazil. During times of convalescence white rice is preferred. Though it has fewer nutrients than brown rice, white rice is easy to digest and will not upset the Stomach or digestion.

Ingredients:
¼ cup coix seed (*yi yi ren*)
1 cup rice (vary black, basmati, jasmine, red, brown, and other types of rice)
2 ½ cups water

Preparation:
1. Rinse rice and coix seed in a colander until water runs clear. If using sweet rice or whole grain rice, soak rice and coix seeds for 8 hours or overnight. If using white rice, break coix seeds into smaller pieces with mortar and pestle to speed cooking time.
2. Place ingredients in a saucepan and bring to a boil. Let simmer 20 minutes for white rice and 60 minutes for whole grain.
3. Turn off heat and let stand 5 minutes.
4. Alternately can be prepared in rice cooker. Use a rice cooker cup and measurement line for proportions of grains to water. It is easier to make sweet rice in a rice cooker as it will get very sticky.

How to Eat:
Eat with paired with vegetables and protein.

Stir-Fried Sticky Rice

Comments:
Sweet (sticky or glutinous) rice has a stronger action to tonify Qi and Blood than other varieties, but it can also cause Phlegm-Damp. If eaten excessively it can cause bloating and indigestion.

Ingredients:
¾ cup sweet (glutinous) rice
5 shitake mushrooms, dried or fresh
2 large pieces dried black wood ear mushroom (hei mu er)
1 carrot, chopped
1 clove of garlic, minced
½ inch ginger, grated or chopped
1 tsp black sesame oil
1 ½ cups of water
dash of rice wine (or sherry)

Preparation:
1. Wash rice and rinse. Soak rice for 8 hours or overnight. Strain.
2. Soak dried mushrooms and wood ear until soft. Discard stem and chop into small pieces.
3. Add sesame oil to frying pan over medium-high heat. Add ginger and garlic. Sauté until browned.
4. Add carrot, mushrooms, and wood ear. Sauté until it has some color and remove.
5. Add more sesame oil to frying pan and sauté rice.
6. Add water and rice wine.
7. Place all ingredients into rice cooker or crockpot and cook for 6 hours.

How to Eat:
Eat 1-2 small bowls daily.

Vegetables

In the traditional Taiwanese postpartum diet, there were no vegetables during the first week. They were considered excessively cooling and clearing. In the second week, red and orange vegetables such as beets, carrots, tomatoes, yams, winter squash, red radishes, and red-tinged greens were introduced to tonify Qi and Blood. Only beginning the third week were vegetables, and some fruit, included in larger amounts. In the modern practice of postpartum recovery this is considered unhealthy. Eat cooked vegetables with every meal. Favor particularly the tonifying vegetables: dark leafy greens, sweet potatoes or yams, carrots, and beets. Vegetables can be incorporated in soups, steamed, steam fried, or sautéed with ginger and black sesame oil. Naturally pickled vegetables can be incorporated, however be careful of salt content. Avoid salads and raw fruit during the first two weeks postpartum as they are too cooling. Beginning the third week add a serving of raw fruit or vegetables if desired. If you are running hot, first try increasing the proportion of cooked vegetables. Then add some raw vegetable and fruit.

Watercress Steam Fry

Comments:
This is an example of a vegetable steam fry to nourish Blood. I got the idea of steam frying from Shelley Young, of the pH Miracle.

Ingredients:
1 bunch watercress, chopped
1 carrot, chopped
½ small onion, chopped
½ inch fresh ginger, chopped
dash of white pepper
a little water to cook

Preparation:
1. Place a frying pan with ¼ inch of water over medium-high heat. Add onions, ginger, and carrots. Sauté 5-10 minutes until carrots are tender. Add more water as needed to keep from drying out.
2. Add watercress and stir. Cook until greens have wilted.

How to Eat:
Eat as a side dish.

Sautéed Beets and Greens

Comments:
This is an example of sautéed vegetables to nourish Blood.

Ingredients:
4-6 beets with green tops
1 bunch Swiss chard
½ small onion, chopped
½ inch fresh ginger, chopped
1 tsp. black sesame oil
dash of white pepper
dash of rice wine

Preparation:

1. Clean and peel beets. Remove the green tops and chop coarsely. Set the green tops aside in a bowl. Slice beets into ¼ inch rounds.
2. Clean and chop Swiss chard. Toss into bowl with the beet green tops
3. Add black sesame oil to a sauce pan over med-high heat. Add ginger and shallots. Sauté until browned.
4. Add beets. Reduce heat and cover.
5. About 10 minutes later when beets become tender, add greens and stir. Add rice wine and cover. Cook until greens have wilted.

How to Eat:

Eat as a side dish.

Sautéed Eggplant[17]

Comments:

Eggplant moves blood, especially in the uterus.

Ingredients:

3 Chinese eggplants or 2 regular eggplants, cubed or cut into strips as preferred

¼ cup peanuts

2 tbsp. soy sauce

2 tbsp. rice vinegar

2 tbsp. rice wine or dry sherry

½ inch fresh ginger, grated

1 clove garlic, minced

safflower or black sesame oil to coat pan

Preparation:

1. Mix soy sauce, vinegar, and wine in a bowl and set aside.
2. Coat a large frying pan with oil and place over medium-high heat. Add ginger and garlic and sauté until they begin to brown. Add peanuts and sauté 1 minute. Add eggplant and sauté until browned.
3. Add sauce mixture and bring to a boil. Lower heat to a simmer, cover, and cook 5-10 minutes until eggplant is cooked.

How to Eat:

Eat as a side dish with any meal.

---

17. Adapted from Young, Grace. "Eggplant in Garlic Sauce." *The Wisdom of the Chinese Kitchen; Classic Family Recipes for Celebration and Healing.* (New York: Simon & Schuster Editions, 1999), 95.

Liver Recipes

Liver is the ideal food during postpartum as it quickly recovers the body from blood loss. Pork liver is traditionally used. It has a neutral thermal temperature, is more bitter than other types of liver, and has the added benefit of reducing edema. In the U.S., this may be difficult to procure. It is most important that the liver be organic and humanely raised. In my opinion, pork liver is the least palatable and chicken liver is the best tasting of the livers. Chicken liver is hot in nature and best suited to those with cold and Yang deficiency, while beef or calves' liver is neutral and benefits the eyes. Choose liver that is soft, elastic, and thick. Eating liver will be the biggest hurdle for most women, and yet it is the best food to both build your Blood and move old Blood out of the body.

Cooking:

To remove strong taste and toxins, soak liver in water with citrus juice (lemon, lime, orange, or calamondin), vinegar, or milk for 30 minutes prior to cooking. Black sesame oil is the traditional oil used in cooking, however butter can cover up the liver taste better. I also like to add peas, onions, and strong spices. Another tip is to put liver in the freezer for 15-30 minutes before cutting it. Thawed liver is slippery and difficult to handle. These are the two ways I deal with the texture issue.

1. I cut the liver in larger "steaks," about 1 ½ inches thick, so that I can sauté them with the outside seared and the middle still pink. This creates a crunchy/creamy experience. The nice seared crust is achieved by a combination of first warming the black sesame oil to high heat before adding the liver to the pan. Dusting the liver first with cornstarch or arrowroot powder mixture prior to frying makes it even better.
2. I cook the liver thoroughly then mash it up into tiny pieces that disappear into the seasoning. You can also ask your butcher to grind it for you.

Ginger:

Use fresh mature ginger as you would find in most supermarkets. Dried ginger is very warming and goes to the Kidneys. Fresh ginger releases the exterior and harmonizes the Spleen and Stomach. When charred, ginger astringes bleeding. When browned (not blackened) it has a specific function as a guiding herb to the uterus and helps to move stagnant Blood there. To brown ginger, slice thinly and fry on each side until it crinkles and browns. It will become more fragrant.

Chinese Rice Wine:

Alcohol is warming and helps move the Blood. Rice wine has a stronger alcohol content than beer or grape wine, and is more akin to dry sherry. Omit if you run hot or have liver issues.

The best way to get ideas for cooking liver is to look at traditional recipes. The following are some basic liver recipes to get you started:

Traditional Taiwanese Recovery Liver Soup[18]

Comments:

This recipe is an authentic postpartum dish. It will be difficult to get compliance with all but the most hardcore postpartum women. Firstly, pork liver has a more bitter flavor than other types of liver. Secondly, there is not enough going on in this recipe to distract the eater from the liver. It builds Blood, breaks up Blood stagnation in the uterus, and helps discharge lochia.

Ingredients (1 day's dosage):
500-700g (1-1.5 lbs.) organic pork liver
citrus juice or vinegar to cover the liver
40g fresh ginger
1 tsp. black sesame oil
2 ½ cups rice wine or Zuo Yue Zi water

Preparation:
1. Rinse liver and soak in citrus juice, milk, or vinegar for 30 minutes. Drain and put in freezer for 15-30 minutes.
2. Remove from freezer and cut into 1cm cubes.
3. Clean ginger and cut into thin pieces.
4. Pour sesame oil into wok or frying pan and put over high heat.
5. Lower to low heat. Add ginger and cook until browned on both sides, but not blackened.
6. Raise heat up to high. Add liver and sauté until it changes color. It is done when it is seared on the outside but is still soft when pressed with a fork.
7. Add rice wine and quickly bring to a boil. Eat while still warm.

How to Eat:
Divide into 2 dosages. Eat the first bowl at breakfast and the second at lunch as the main dish. It can be paired with Yi Ren Rice or congee.

Simple Liver & Onions

Comments:

This is perhaps the best known way to eat liver. Builds Blood and helps discharge lochia.

Ingredients:
17-25 oz. (1-1.5 lbs.) organic liver
citrus juice or vinegar to cover the liver
½ inch fresh ginger, finely chopped
1 medium onion, chopped
any flour or cornstarch to coat liver

---

18. Adapted from Shuqi Zhuang. *Postpartum Recovery Program; a Manual of Rules and Recipes for the Postpartum Woman.* (Taiwan: Guang He Chu Ban She, 2005). ISBN 9578807015

1 tsp. black sesame oil
(optional) a little sausage or bacon for flavor
dash of rice wine, dry sherry, or red wine
1 tsp. each: cumin, sage, thyme, and rosemary

Preparation:
1. Rinse liver and soak in citrus juice, milk, or vinegar for 30 minutes. Drain. If you want to cut into smaller pieces, put in the freezer for 15 minutes to make it easier to handle. Then remove and cut into ½ inch cubes or tiny pieces. Otherwise, leave whole (chicken livers) or in large steaks and proceed to the next step.
2. Place flour in a bowl. Season with pepper. Toss in liver and coat. Remove each coated piece of liver and place on a plate.
3. Pour sesame oil into a frying pan and put over high heat. Add onions and ginger and cook until browned. Add herbs and spices.
4. Add liver and brown on both sides. Add a generous dash of alcohol. (Add sausage or bacon if using). Cover and simmer for a few minutes. It is done when it is seared on the outside but is still soft when pressed with a fork. Serve warm.

How to Eat:
This recipe can be paired with Yi Ren Rice and vegetables.

Jacquie's Savory Chopped Liver[19]

Comments:
Jewish communities in the U.S. are one of the few places where you will still find people eating liver and actually enjoying it. Jacquie learned to make the traditional chopped chicken liver from her grandmother "who chopped it with a 5-bladed hand chopper in a big wooden bowl", and then modified grandma's recipe to appeal to liver-averse friends. Her modifications: broil the livers till they are thoroughly browned on both sides, almost caramelized. Omit the matzo meal or other starch. Sauté the onion in a minimum of olive oil, again until caramelized or almost that cooked, and add a good soy sauce right at the end. When dealing with a difficult flavor you cannot mask, the best strategy is to add another strong flavor to take it in a new direction. This recipe builds Blood and helps discharge lochia.

Ingredients:
17-25 oz. (1-1.5 lbs.) organic chicken livers
1 medium onion, chopped
2-4 eggs
garlic granules or powder to taste

---

19. Jacquie Lowell teaches creative thinking and improvisational comedy in San Diego, and directs Outside the Lines improv comedy performing troupe. She enjoys creative cooking, and suggests that "a chopped liver sculpture on the buffet table can be comedy theater as well as delicious."

your favorite soy sauce to taste
olive oil to coat pan for sautéing onions

Preparation:

1. Put the eggs in a pot of water to boil until hard boiled, drain, peel and let cool.
2. Rinse livers, and spread out evenly in a toaster-oven pan. Broil until dark brown and crispy on both sides, but remove before the edges char. Let cool. Alternately, you can broil them in a standard oven at 425°F.
3. Slice the onion and sauté in a minimum of oil until the pieces become limp and fragrant, even until caramelized. Then add the soy sauce and cook a bit more.
4. Put all ingredients (cooked eggs, livers and onions, plus garlic) in a large bowl and mash together thoroughly with a fork, or well-washed hands, or use a food processor if you want an even smoother texture. Add additional garlic or soy sauce to taste.

How to Eat:

Enjoy on the cracker of your choice. Traditionally, chopped liver is eaten on matzoh (a basic wheat and water cracker), but goes well with any crackers. Optional: garnish with a leaf of parsley, baby spinach, cilantro, or other favorite green.

Liver Ragu[20]

Comments:

Noodles and peas disguise much of the liver experience. Builds Blood and helps discharge lochia.

Ingredients (1 day's dosage):

17-25 ounces (1-1.5 lbs.) organic liver
citrus juice or vinegar to cover the liver
8 ounce bag noodles of your choice
4 ounce bag of frozen peas
1 cup leafy greens (spinach, kale, etc.), chopped
½ inch fresh ginger, finely chopped
1 onion, chopped
1 small clove garlic, minced
1 tsp. each: tarragon, thyme, marjoram
1 bunch parsley, chopped
olive oil and butter to coat pan
4 cups soup stock
dash of rice wine or dry wine

> **A POTENT BLOOD TONIC**
>
> My grandfather was an OBGYN in Rio de Janeiro, Brazil. I remember hearing how they used to serve liver in the hospital to patients who were anemic. Until a generation ago liver was a commonly eaten food in most households. Unfortunately, now outside of Jewish or certain ethnic communities, it is a rare occurrence. I have witnessed countless times how a week of eating liver can quickly recover a patient from even severe blood loss. When blood tonics and astringent herbs are also used the results are incredible.

20. Adapted from Debra Mayhew. *The Soup Bible.* (New York: Barnes & Noble Inc., 2006), 251.

Preparation:

1. Rinse liver and soak in citrus juice, milk, or vinegar for 30 minutes. Drain and put in freezer for 15-30 minutes. Remove liver from freezer and chop into small pieces.

2. Coat a medium to large saucepan with oil and butter and place over high heat. Add onions and ginger and sauté until browned. Add garlic, herbs, then liver. Brown liver evenly but leave undercooked. Add rice wine. Remove liver from pot and place in a bowl. At this point you can break the liver up into even small pieces that will disappear in the soup, if desired.

3. Add soup stock to the same saucepan. Bring to a boil and add pasta. Cook until pasta is cooked (typically 5-8 minutes). Add peas, parsley, peas, and greens. Simmer until they change color and become vibrant green.

4. Add liver and remove from heat. Serve warm.

How to Eat:

Eat a bowl for lunch or dinner as a complete meal.

Gordon's Scottish Meatloaf

Comments:

This recipe is a take on haggis, inspired by a conversation with a homesick Scotsman, Gordon Kelly. He also suggested modifying mince and tatties, another famous Scottish dish as it also included strong flavors to drown out the liver. Builds Blood and help discharge lochia.

Ingredients:

1 lb. organic liver

lime juice, milk, or vinegar to soak liver

1 lb. beef, any cut you like

½ lb. steel cut (Irish) or Scottish (finer ground) oats

3 carrots, finely chopped

3 medium onions, finely chopped

1 inch fresh ginger, finely chopped

½ tsp. each: nutmeg, black or white pepper, mustard powder[21]

2 eggs

butter to coat pan

½ cup dark beer or soup stock

Preparation:

1. Rinse liver and soak in citrus juice, milk, or vinegar for 30 minutes. Drain and put in freezer for 15-30 minutes. Remove liver from freezer and chop into tiny pieces. Chop beef into in very small pieces.

---

21. Other traditional haggis spices include: clove, nutmeg, coriander, allspice, and cayenne pepper. Experiment to find your preferred mix.

2. (Optional) For a more authentic taste, place oats on a cooking sheet and toast in a 350° oven for 20 minutes, stirring as necessary to keep from burning.
3. Coat a medium saucepan with butter and place over high heat. Add onions and ginger. Sauté until browned. Add spices, then meat and sauté until browned but not thoroughly cooked. Remove from heat and add oats, carrots, and beer or stock. Scramble eggs and add.
4. Preheat oven to 350°. Coat a baking pan with butter. Add contents from pot and bake for 20 minutes. Remove from oven and serve warm.

How to Eat:
Eat a bowl for lunch or dinner with mashed potatoes and steamed vegetables.

Liver Laab[22]

Comments:
This is a Thai/Laoation-style recipe where liver is substituted for ground pork. I love how the Scottish and Thai people came to similar conclusions of using toasted grain, strong spices, and small pieces to disguise organ meats. Builds Blood and help discharge lochia.

Ingredients:
½ lb. organic liver, ground or cut into tiny pieces
¼ lb. organic ground beef or pork
3 tbsp. soy sauce
2 limes
1 scallion, thinly chopped
½ inch fresh ginger, finely chopped
¼ tsp. ground chili powder (optional)
5 sprigs of cilantro, chopped
3 sprigs of mint, chopped
1 tbsp. uncooked rice
vegetable oil to coat pan salt to taste
dash of rice wine

Preparation:
1. Rinse liver and soak in citrus juice, milk, or vinegar for 30 minutes. Drain. If liver is not ground, put in freezer for 15-30 minutes. Remove liver from freezer and cut into tiny pieces.
2. Add oil to frying pan over medium-high heat. Add rice and sauté until browned but not blackened. Cool and pulse through a food processor until coarsely chopped. Conserve.

22. Adapted from (2012). *Laab*. Retrieved from www.thaitable.com/thai/recipe/pork-rice-porridge

3. Add oil to frying pan over medium-high heat. Add ginger and sauté until browned. Add liver and sauté until cooked.

4. In a bowl, mix soy sauce, toasted rice, lime juice to taste, chili powder, scallion, mint, rice wine, and cilantro. Add liver and ginger. Mix well.

How to Eat:
Eat with sticky rice, Yi Ren Rice, or congee.

Portuguese-Style Liver with Potatoes[23]

Comments:
My mom grew up in a Portuguese neighborhood in Rio de Janeiro. For liver, she recommends a traditional Portuguese dish, Iscas Lisboetas. It builds Blood and help discharge lochia.

Ingredients:
17-25 ounces (1-1.5 lbs.) organic beef liver
potatoes for boiling
butter and olive oil to coat the pan
for Marinade:
2/3 cup of rice wine or sherry
1 tbsp. olive oil
1 tbsp. chopped scallions
1 tbsp. fresh ginger, grated
juice and zest of 1 lime
2 bay leaves
1 clove garlic, minced (omit if have Heat signs)
black or white pepper to taste

Preparation:
1. **The day before:** Rinse liver and put in the freezer for 15-30 minutes. Remove from freezer and cut liver into very thin slices.
2. Mix the marinade ingredients. Place liver in a glass container. Cover with marinade mixture. Make sure each piece of liver is fully coated. Cover and place in refrigerator overnight.
3. **The next day:** Bring a pot of water to a boil. Wash the potatoes and add them whole. Cook until potatoes are soft. Drain. When cool enough to handle, peel them and cut in medium thick slices. Cover and keep warm.
4. Meanwhile, remove liver from marinade and let dry a bit on a plate. Conserve marinade.
5. Heat butter and olive oil in a frying pan over medium heat. Skim some of the ginger, scallions, and herbs from the marinade and sauté in the pan for 2 minutes. Bring to high

---

23. Based on my mom, Dr. Judith Andrews', recipe.

heat and add liver. Fry until browned on both sides but still undercooked and soft (about 5 minutes each side). Remove the liver and keep warm.

6. Add the marinade to the pan, bring to a boil and allow the alcohol to evaporate and the sauce to reduce.
7. Serve immediately the liver and potatoes on a plate covered with the sauce.

How to Eat:
Eat with steamed vegetables.

Liver with Wine Sauce Reduction[24]

Comments:
This recipe adds a starchy coating to the liver and a flavorful sauce. It builds Blood and help discharge lochia.

Sauce Ingredients:
butter to coat pan
1 cup mushrooms, sliced
½ cup carrots, sliced
½ cup shallots, sliced
8 sprigs parsley
2 sprigs thyme
½ inch fresh ginger, thinly chopped
1 cup rice wine or sherry
4 cups soup stock

Sauté Ingredients:
butter to coat the pan
17-25 ounces (1-1.5 lbs.) organic liver
cornstarch, arrowroot powder, or tapioca starch to coat liver
white or black pepper to taste

Preparation:
Sauce:
1. Heat bone stock to a simmer.
2. Heat butter or oil in a large sauce pan over medium heat. Add ginger and sauté until browned, but not blackened. Add vegetables and herbs. Sauté for another 2 minutes until they change color and become more vibrant.
3. Add bone stock to pot. Simmer uncovered until it reduces to about 1 cup. Strain sauce and conserve.

---

24. Adapted from Thomas Keller. *The French Laundry Cookbook.* (New York: Artisan, 1999).

Liver:

1. Rinse liver and soak in citrus juice, milk, or vinegar for 30 minutes. Drain. If liver is not ground, put in freezer for 15 minutes to firm up. Remove liver from freezer and cut into ½ inch steaks or tiny pieces. Coat in starch. Season with pepper.
2. Coat frying pan with butter and place over high heat. Add liver and reduce to medium heat. Cook each side about 5 minutes. Liver should look browned, have a firm yet springy give to it. Remove. You may want to sauté some greens to go with it.
3. Place liver on a plate and cover with sauce.

How to Eat:
Eat with Yi Ren Rice, potatoes, or congee and vegetables.

Pirão de Fígado

Comments:

Manioc flour[25] is the fiber left over when the juice is extracted from the manioc tuber to make tapioca. It is eaten toasted throughout Brazil paired with rice and beans. In Northeastern Brazil manioc flour is added as a thickening agent to flavorful sauces to make what is called "pirão." Manioc flour not only adds texture to disguise the liver, it is also wonderful for regulating bowel movements without side effects.

Ingredients:

17-25 ounces (1-1.5 lbs.) organic liver
1 cup manioc flour
1 cup collard greens (or other greens of your choice), finely chopped
2 medium tomatoes, chopped
1 small onion, finely chopped
½ inch fresh ginger, grated
Several sprigs of parsley or cilantro, finely chopped
½ clove garlic, minced (omit if have Heat signs)
1 cup soup stock
dash of rice wine, sherry, or white wine (optional)
butter and olive oil to coat the pan

Preparation:

1. Rinse liver and soak in citrus juice, milk, or vinegar for 30 minutes. Drain. If liver is not ground, put in freezer for 15 minutes. Remove liver from freezer and cut into tiny pieces.
2. Add oil to saucepan and bring to high heat. Add onions, ginger, and garlic and sauté until they begin to brown.
3. Add liver and brown on both sides. Remove liver from heat and keep warm.

---

25. Manioc flour can be purchased at Brazilian grocery stores and online retailers. It is also goes by: farinha de mandioca, cassava flour, or yucca flour.

4. Do not clean the saucepan before adding greens and tomatoes and returning to medium-high flame. Add manioc flour. Sauté for a minute or so.

5. Add soup stock, wine, and parsley. Bring to a simmer stirring constantly. Reincorporate liver. Cook until it thickens.

How to Eat:
Eat with Yi Ren Rice or congee.

Liver Paprikash[26]

Comments:
Paprikash, most famously made of chicken, is a Hungarian dish with a heavy dose of paprika. Paprika is ground chili peppers and is a powerful flavor that partners well with organ meats.

Ingredients:
17-25 ounces (1-1.5 lbs.) organic liver (the original recipe calls for pork or lamb)
2 organic lamb or pork hearts (optional)
vinegar or citrus juice to soak livers
2 onions, finely chopped
1 inch piece fresh ginger, finely chopped
1 tbsp. sweet paprika
1 tbsp. smoked paprika (or Spanish pimentón, optional)
2 tsp. hot paprika (optional)
8 ounces tomato passata[27]
1 bunch parsley, chopped
sea salt and freshly ground black pepper to taste
dash of wine
½ cup sour cream (optional)
olive oil and butter to coat pan

Preparation:
1. Rinse liver and soak in citrus juice, milk, or vinegar for 30 minutes. Drain. If liver is not ground, put in freezer for 15 minutes. Remove liver from freezer and cut into large pieces.

2. Cut the hearts in half lengthwise and remove the coarse ventricles. Rinse and pat dry.

3. Coat a saucepan with oil and butter and place over medium-high heat. Add onions and ginger and sauté until browned. Add paprika and stir thoroughly. Add organ meat and sauté until browned.

4. Add passata, a dash of wine, parsley, and a little water. Cover and bring to a simmer.

---

26. Adapted from Hugh-Fearnley Whittingstall. (2013). *Paprikash of hearts and livers.* Retrieved from http://www.theguardian.com/lifeandstyle/2013/apr/19/offal-recipes-whittingstall

27. Tomato passata is uncooked tomato purée that has been strained of seeds and skins. My Italian great-grandmother passed on an aversion to using tomato seeds and skins in cooked recipes, as they contaminate the recipe with bitterness. You can sometimes find passata hiding amongst tomato paste at the supermarket, or else buy canned tomatoes and remove the seeds and skin.

Reduce heat as low as possible. Cook for 2 hours or more until the meat is very tender. Check frequently and add water as necessary.

5. When the sauce is thickened and the meat tender, remove from heat and add sour cream, if desired.

How to Eat:
Traditionally eaten with mashed potaoes, but can also be paired with Yi Ren Rice.

Kidney Recipes

Eating kidneys is powerful medicine during any period of deficiency. In Taiwanese postpartum recovery, kidneys are eaten during the second week to speed metabolism and help contract the uterus. They tonify the Kidneys for issues such as low back pain, low libido, fatigue, etc. They also treat the emotional level: timidity and weak boundaries. However, environmental toxins tend to collect in the kidneys, making it increasingly difficult to get a safe supply. They also require more thorough cleaning than liver. For these reasons many will choose to forgo them. For more recipes, substitute kidney in the liver recipes above.

Cooking:

Properly prepared, some find kidneys more palatable than liver. Be sure to cut them in half and remove all the white membranous material prior to cooking. If not, there will be a distinct urine smell and taste that renders the kidneys inedible. Kidneys should be soaked in citrus (lemon, lime, orange) juice or vinegar to remove toxins and remnants of urine or blood. Prepare them with browned ginger, black sesame oil, and rice wine, as the liver above. Be sure to buy organic kidneys.

Pork kidneys are preferred in traditional Chinese and Taiwanese postpartum recovery due to their neutral thermal temperature. I find them too strong tasting and prefer lamb or beef. Lamb kidneys are the most heating and appropriate for Yang deficiency. Beef kidneys are less warming.

Traditional Taiwanese Recovery Kidney Soup[28]

Comments:
This recipe is an authentic postpartum dish. It will be difficult to get compliance with all but the most hardcore postpartum women. Firstly, pork kidney has a more gamy flavor than other types of kidney. Secondly, there is not enough going on in this recipe to distract the eater from the kidney. Speeds metabolism and helps contract the uterus.

Ingredients :
2 organic pork kidneys

---

28. Adapted from Shuqi Zhuang. *Postpartum Recovery Program; a Manual of Rules and Recipes for the Postpartum Woman.* (Taiwan: Guang He Chu Ban She, 2005). ISBN 9578807015

citrus juice or vinegar to cover kidneys
40g fresh ginger, finely sliced
black sesame oil to coat pan
2 ½ cups rice wine or Zuo Yue Zi water

Preparation:
1. Rinse kidneys. Cut in half. Remove the white-colored membranes (urinary glands). Rinse the kidneys again. Soak in citrus juice or vinegar for 30 minutes. Strain and pat dry.
2. Traditionally, the kidneys are scored in two directions, like graph paper, so that the kidneys form "flowers" when cooked. You may do this, slice them, or leave them halved.
3. Add black sesame oil to frying pan and put over high heat, Add ginger, reduce to low heat. Sauté until ginger is browned on both sides, but not blackened.
4. Turn up to high heat again. Add kidneys and sauté until you see a change in color.
5. Add rice wine and bring to a boil. Turn off heat and serve while still warm.

How to Eat:
Divide into two bowls. It can be paired with a serving of Yi Ren rice.

Steak & Kidney Pie

Comments:
This is a British staple; time consuming but tasty. Speeds metabolism and helps contract the uterus.

Ingredients:
1 ½ lb. beef chuck steak, cut into 1 inch cubes
½ lb. organic kidneys
citrus juice or vinegar to cover kidneys
½ inch fresh ginger, finely sliced
2 onions, finely chopped
3 carrots, diced
2 stalks of celery, diced
½ cup mushrooms, chopped
1 tsp thyme
black or white pepper to taste
1 bay leaf
5 sprigs of parsley, finely chopped
1 clove garlic, minced (omit if Heat signs)
1 tbsp. tomato paste
2 tbsp. Worcestershire sauce
1 egg, beaten
2 tbsp. plain flour or gluten free blend

1 cup (8 ounces) dark beer

1 ½ cups soup stock

butter and olive oill to coat pan

12 ounces puff pastry (2 pieces of dough; 1 to line dish and 1to cover)

Preparation:

1. Rinse kidneys. Cut in half. Remove the white-colored membranes (urinary glands). Rinse the kidneys again. Soak in citrus juice or vinegar for 30 min. Strain and pat dry. Cut kidneys into small pieces.
2. Coat a large saucepan with butter and olive oil and place over medium-high heat. Add onions, ginger, and garlic and sauté until browned.
3. Add beef and kidneys and brown evenly. Add thyme, celery, carrots, and mushrooms and sauté until bright and slightly browned.
4. Reduce to medium heat. Stir in flour. Keep stirring for 2-3 minutes to cook the flour.
5. Add tomato paste, bay leaf, and parsley. Stir. Add beer and soup stock. Bring to a simmer.
6. Skim off bubbles and impurities. Simmer partially covered for 1 ½ hours until the meat is tender.
7. Remove from heat and add Worcestershire sauce.
8. Preheat oven to 425°F. Spread pie crust in a baking dish. Fill with meat mixture and allow to cool until just warm. Cover pie with second piece of dough. Pinch the edges together to seal. Make small cuts to allow steam to escape. Brush the top layer of crust with egg.
9. Place in oven and bake for 30-40 minutes until crust is golden brown.

How to Eat:

Eat a slice as the main dish.

Pirão de Rim

Comments:

Manioc flour[29] is the fiber left over when the juice is extracted from the manioc tuber to make tapioca. It is eaten toasted throughout Brazil paired with rice and beans. In Northeastern Brazil manioc flour is added as a thickening agent to flavorful sauces to make what is called "pirão." Manioc flour not only adds texture to disguise the kidney, it is also wonderful for regulating bowel movements without side effects.

Ingredients:

2 organic kidneys

¼ cup manioc flour

¼ cup parsley, finely chopped

1 medium tomato, chopped

---

29. Manioc flour can be purchased at Brazilian grocery stores and online retailers. It is also goes by: farinha de mandioca, cassava flour, or yucca flour.

1 small onion, finely chopped
½ inch fresh ginger, grated
¼ tsp. each: cumin, paprika, thyme
½ clove garlic, minced (omit if have Heat signs)
1 cup soup stock
dash of rice wine, sherry, or white wine (optional)
butter and olive oil to coat the pan

Preparation:

1. Rinse kidneys and cut in half. Cut out any white, membranous material with cooking scissors. Soak in citrus juice or vinegar for 30 minutes. Drain and rinse. Cut into small pieces.
2. Add oil to saucepan and bring to high heat. Add onions, ginger, and garlic and sauté until they begin to brown. Add spices. Add kidneys and brown on both sides. Add tomato and parsley. Add soup stock and bring to a boil. Simmer for 5-10 minutes until cooked.
3. Add manioc flour stirring constantly. Remove from heat and serve.

How to Eat:

Eat with Yi Ren Rice or congee.

Beef & Kidney Stroganoff

Comments:

Beef stroganoff was a staple in my house growing up. In Brazil, they use crème de leite (or heavy cream) instead of sour cream. This recipe is from my mom's childhood nanny, housekeeper, and family member, Durva.[30] She would probably not be pleased that I added kidneys to it.

Ingredients:

8 ounces beef sirloin, thinly sliced or ground
2 organic kidneys
½ cup mushroom, thinly sliced
2 tomatoes, skin removed and diced
1 small onion, finely chopped
1 tbsp. ketchup
olive oil to coat pan
2-3 tbsp. sour cream, to taste
¼ tsp. each: dill, tarragon

Preparation:

1. Rinse kidneys and cut in half. Cut out any white, membranous material with cooking

---

30. Durva was also a singer and songwriter who had a small following.

scissors. Soak in citrus juice, milk, or vinegar for 30 minutes. Drain and rinse. Cut into small pieces.

2. Add oil to saucepan and bring to high heat. Add onions and sauté until translucent. Add beef and kidneys and brown. Add mushrooms, tomatoes, ketchup, and herbs. Cover and cook for 5-10 until meat is cooked and mushrooms are soft.

3. Remove from heat. Add sour cream and stir thoroughly. Serve warm.

How to Eat:
Eat with Yi Ren Rice or congee.

Devilled Kidneys on Toast[31]

Comments:
This English recipe covers the taste of kidney with strong flavors.

Ingredients:
4 organic kidneys
vinegar or citrus juice to soak kidneys
olive oil to coat pan
4 ounces rice wine or sherry
1 tsp. red currant jelly (can substitute raspberry jelly)
1 tbsp. Worcestershire sauce
pinch of cayenne pepper
1 tbsp. mustard
Sea salt and freshly ground black pepper
1 tbsp. heavy cream
parsley, chopped, for garnish

Preparation:
1. Rinse kidneys and cut in half. Cut out any white, membranous material with cooking scissors. Soak in citrus juice or vinegar for 30 minutes. Drain and rinse. Cut into small pieces.

2. Coat a saucepan with oil and place over medium-high heat. Add kidneys and sauté until browned. Add rice wine.

3. Stir in jelly, Worcestershire sauce, cayenne pepper, mustard, and black pepper to taste. Add a pinch of salt and cream. Bring to a simmer and cook for a few minutes, stirring, until the sauce is reduced and thickened. Remove from heat.

How to Eat:
Serve on toast, with parsley scattered on top.

---

31. Adapted from Hugh-Fearnley Whittingstall. (2013). *Deviled kidneys on toas*t. Retrieved from http://www.theguardian.com/lifeandstyle/2013/apr/19/offal-recipes-whittingstall

Chicken Recipes

Beginning the third week postpartum the body is strong enough to assimilate strong tonics. Chicken is an important Qi and Blood tonic and should be eaten regularly for a full six months after giving birth (or for the duration of breastfeeding). Doing so will promote adequate milk production, as well as build good health in both mother and baby.

Traditional Taiwanese Recovery Chicken[32]

Comments:
The use of alcohol will seem excessive to most Westerners. This recipe tonifies Qi and Blood.

Ingredients (1 day's dosage):
approximately half a chicken[33]
½ inch fresh ginger, chopped
black sesame oil to coat pan
2 ½ cups rice wine or Zuo Yue Zi water

Preparation:
1. Rinse the chicken, then cut into small pieces.
2. Add black sesame oil to a sauce pan and place over medium-high heat. Add ginger and sauté until it browned, but not blackened.
3. Add chicken and sauté for 7 minutes, or until cooked through.
4. Add rice wine. Cover pot and bring to a boil. Reduce heat and simmer for 15-20 minutes.

How to Eat:
This recipe can be paired with Yi Ren Rice and vegetables.

Sautéed Ginger Chicken

Comments:
A basic recipe to tonify Qi and Blood.

Ingredients:
2 breasts or 4 thighs organic chicken
1 inch fresh ginger, finely chopped
4 scallion stalks, chopped
1 tsp. black sesame oil
generous dash of rice wine, dry sherry, or red wine

---

32. Adapted from Shuqi Zhuang. *Postpartum Recovery Program; a Manual of Rules and Recipes for the Postpartum Woman.* (Taiwan: Guang He Chu Ban She, 2005). ISBN 9578807015

33. Note, American-grown chickens are much stouter than Asian chickens. A chicken breast is sufficient.

Preparation:
1. Rinse chicken, remove skin, and pat dry.
2. Pour sesame oil into a frying pan and put over high heat. Add ginger and cook until browned.
3. Add chicken and brown on both sides. Add a generous dash of wine. Cover and simmer until fully cooked. Serve warm.

How to Eat:
This recipe can be paired with Yi Ren Rice and vegetables.

Calamondin Roast Chicken

Ingredients:
1 small chicken
1 bunch of thyme, tarragon, parsley, finely chopped
1 clove garlic, minced
½ an onion, finely chopped
½ inch fresh ginger, grated
1 tbsp. black sesame oil
6 calamondins (can substitute komquats or tangerines), sliced
black or white pepper as desired

Preparation:
1. Preheat oven to 350° F.
2. Bring a large pot of water to a boil. Blanch chicken for 2 minutes. Remove the chicken and drain.
3. Place chicken in baking pan. Mix black sesame oil, herbs, onions, garlic, and ginger in a bowl. Apply the oil mixture to the entire chicken. Squeeze calamondin slices over the chicken and place on top of chicken.
4. Place in the oven. Cover when it begins to brown. Cook 45-60 minutes.

How to Eat:
Pair with Yi Ren Rice and steamed vegetables.

Dang Gui Chicken Soup

Comments:
This is a traditional Chinese recipe to strongly recover from blood loss and is typically eaten after menses is over.

Ingredients:
1 black chicken (silkie chicken, can substitute regular chicken)
packet of Chinese herbs from TCM herbalist (includes Chinese angelica (dang gui))
1 inch fresh ginger, sliced
1 bottle rice wine
water to cover

Preparation:
1. Bring a big saucepan full of water to a boil. Add chicken and boil for 5 minutes. Strain and discard water.
2. Rinse herbs. Add ingredients to a large saucepan or crockpot and simmer 8 hours or overnight.
3. Remove chicken and mince. Strain broth. Add chicken meat back to stock. Discard herbs and chicken bones Serve warm.

How to Eat:
Eat a bowl as a complete meal.

Vegan Lunch Recipes

Seitan Noodle Bowl[34]

Comments:
A nourishing vegan dish.

Ingredients:
8 ounces seitan, cut into cubes
1 carrot, chopped
½ cup broccoli, chopped
¼ cup raw peanuts
8 ounce package soba noodles
1 tbsp. tamari or soy sauce
1 tbsp. teriyaki sauce
1 tbsp. rice wine or dry sherry
1 scallion stalk, finely chopped
1 tsp. fresh ginger, finely chopped
1 clove garlic, finely chopped (omit if Heat signs)
black sesame oil to coat pan

> **VEGAN TIP**
>
> Vegans and vegetarians can render food more warming and nourishing by roasting and slow cooking. Adding food herbs boosts a recipe's ability to tonify Qi and Blood.

---

34. Adapted from Tendollarwine. (2007). *Vegan Seitan Noodle Bowl*. Retrieved from www.food.com/recipe/vegan-seitan-noodle-bowl-272850

Preparation:

1. Coat frying pan with oil and place over medium-high heat. Add ginger and garlic and sauté until they begin to brown and become fragrant. Add seitan and peanuts and sauté until they begin to brown. Add carrots and broccoli and sauté for 1 minute.

2. Add sauces, wine, and scallions and bring to a simmer. When vegetable are cooked remove from heat.

3. Meanwhile, fill a medium saucepan with water and a little salt and vegetable oil and bring to a rolling boil. Add soba noodles and boil until noodles are cooked to your liking. When noodles are done, strain.

4. Place a serving of noodles in a bowl and top with seitan vegetable mixture. Serve.

How to Eat:

Eat as main course for lunch or dinner.

Tempeh Tikka Masala[35]

Comments:

A nourishing vegan dish.

Ingredients:

Tempeh marinade:

4 oz. tempeh cut into small cubes (can substitute firm tofu or seitan)

½ cup water

½ tsp. garam masala

½ tsp paprika

1 tsp Greek yogurt or non-dairy substitute

oil to coat pan

Curry:

½ tsp. garam masala

¼ tsp. paprika

1 tsp. coriander

pinch of asafetida (hing, optional)

1 tsp. turmeric

1 small onion, finely chopped

½ cup kale or other greens, finely chopped

3 medium tomatoes, chopped

1 inch fresh ginger, finely chopped

1 clove garlic, minced

½ tsp raw sugar (optional)

---

35. Adapted from Lysa. (2012). *Tempeh Tikka Masala with Kale*. Retrieved from www.veganricha.com/2012/05/tempeh-tikka-masala-with-kale-vegan.html

2 tbsp. plain Greek yogurt or non-dairy substitute

3-5 tbsp. whole milk, or almond or hemp milk

oil to coat pan

Preparation:

1. Mix all the ingredients of the marinade and add tempeh. Place tempeh and marinade in a small sauce pan and place over low heat until liquid has absorbed (about 15-20 minutes). Add a little oil to coat the saucepan and sauté tempeh until it browns on both sides. Remove from heat and put side.

2. Blend tomatoes in a blender until thoroughly puréed.

3. Coat a medium saucepan with oil and place over medium-high heat. Add onions, ginger, and garlic and sauté until browned but not blackened. Add spices and sauté for 1 minute.

4. Add greens and sauté. Add tomato purée and cook on medium-low heat for 15-20 minutes stirring occasionally, until the mix thickens.

5. Add tempeh, yogurt, and sugar and mix thoroughly. Slowly add milk until you reach the consistency you prefer. Mix well and bring to a boil over low heat. Remove from heat and serve warm.

How to Eat:

Pair with Yi Ren Rice.

Palak Tempeh[36]

Comments:

Spinach and dark leafy greens build Blood.

Ingredients:

4 oz. tempeh cut into small cubes (can substitute firm tofu or seitan)

3 cups spinach (or other greens), chopped

2 tomatoes, chopped

1 small onion, finely chopped

1 inch fresh ginger, finely chopped

1 clove garlic, minced (omit if Heat signs)

½ tsp. raw sugar (optional)

pinch of asafetida (hing, optional)

1 tsp. turmeric

¼ tsp cinnamon, clove, nutmeg, and cardamom

1 bay leaf

2 tbsp. peanuts

---

36. Adapted from Lysa. (2014). *Palak Tempeh*. Retrieved from www.veganricha.com/2011/07/palak-tempehtempeh-in-spinach-tomato.html

ghee to coat pan
water

Preparation:

1. Soak peanuts in water for 1 hour.
2. Blend spinach and tomatoes in a blender until thoroughly pureed. Pour into a bowl and put aside.
3. Blend peanuts with a little water until thoroughly puréed. Pour into a bowl and conserve.
4. Coat medium saucepan with ghee and place over medium heat. Add onion, ginger, and garlic. Sauté until browned but not blackened.
5. Add spices and sauté. Add tempeh and sauté until browned.
6. Add spinach and tomato purée and sugar and mix thoroughly. Simmer over low heat for 20-30 minutes until it thickens.
7. Add peanut puree. Slowly add water until it reaches your preferred consistency. Bring to a boil over medium heat. Remove from heat and serve warm.

How to Eat:
Pair with Yi Ren Rice.

Thai Curry Squash[37]

Comments:
This is a warming, nourishing vegan recipe.

Ingredients:
1 medium kabocha squash (or winter squash), cut into 1-inch cubes
2 large tomatoes, chopped
1 medium onion, chopped
½ inch fresh ginger, grated
1 clove garlic, minced (optional, if no Heat signs)
1 tbsp. Thai red curry paste
13- to 14-ounce can coconut milk
½ cup water
1 tbsp. soy sauce
juice from 1 lime
1 bunch cilantro, chopped
oil to coat pan

Preparation:

1. Coat a large saucepan with oil and place over medium-high heat. Add onions, then ginger

---

37. Adapted from Lavery, Lisa. (2012). *Thai Red Curry with Kabocha Squash*. Retrieved from www.chow.com/recipes/30268-thai-red-curry-with-kabocha-squash

and garlic and sauté until browned. Add curry paste and sauté 1 minute. Add squash and sauté 1 minute.

2. Add coconut milk, water, soy sauce, and tomatoes. Bring to a boil, then lower heat to a simmer. Simmer for 30 minutes. Remove from heat and add lime juice and cilantro.

How to Eat:
Eat warm over Yi Ren Rice.

Polenta Lasagna[38]

Comments:
This dish is the perfect comfort food. Eggplant moves Blood. Spinach builds Blood. Lentils and cheese provide protein. Whole grain cornmeal provides fiber.

Ingredients:
Polenta:
2 cups whole grain cornmeal
6 cups water or soup broth

Lasagna:
1 eggplant, sliced length-wise in medium-thin strips
1 jar pasta sauce
6 mushrooms, sliced
1 clove garlic, chopped
2 tbsp. water
10 oz. package frozen spinach
1 cup cooked lentils
2 cups of shredded mozzarella (or cheese substitute)
pepper to taste
olive oil to coat pan

Preparation:
1. Make the polenta ahead of time: Add water to a large saucepan and place over medium high heat. Bring to a boil. Slowly whisk in cornmeal. Keep whisking to avoid clumping. Reduce heat to low and cook until cornmeal thickens (about 15 minutes). Remove from heat. Pour the polenta into a 9 x 13 dish and smooth the top. Allow it to cool in the refrigerator for at least an hour.
2. Once set, cut the polenta into ½ inch strips and set aside.
3. Coat a large frying pan with olive oil and place over medium high heat. Add 2 or 3 eggplant

---

38. Adapted from Not Crocker. (2012). *Mushroom and Eggplant Polenta Lasagna.* Retrieved from www. notcrocker. com/2012/05/05/mushroom-and-eggplant-polenta-lasagna

strips and sauté on each side until browned. Set aside and repeat with more strips, until all the eggplant is cooked. Set eggplant strips aside.

4. Add more olive oil to the frying pan and return to heat. Add garlic, pepper, mushrooms, and spinach. Sauté until mushrooms change color. Remove from heat and set aside.

5. In a medium bowl mash lentils and ½ cup of cheese. Add sautéed spinach and mushrooms and mix well.

6. Preheat oven to 375°. Coat the bottom of a casserole dish with pasta sauce. Place a layer of polenta strips over the sauce, leaving a little space in between them. Cover with more sauce. Place a layer of eggplant strips. Cover with more sauce. Sprinkle a layer of cheese. Place a second layer of polenta. Spread spinach/lentil mixture. Place a second layer of eggplant. Sprinkle a final layer of cheese.

7. Cover the dish with aluminum foil. Place in the oven and bake covered for 30 minutes. Then remove foil and bake an additional 20 minutes. Let stand 10 minutes before serving.

How to Eat:
Eat a serving for lunch or dinner.

3 Bean Salad

Comments:
This recipe is perfect if you are running warm. Be sure to serve it slightly warmed and not cold.

Ingredients:
½ cup adzuki beans, canned or pre-cooked
½ cup black beans, canned or pre-cooked
½ cup green beans, canned or pre-cooked, thinly sliced
2 scallions, finely chopped
1 small bunch parsley, finely chopped
½ tbsp. black sesame oil
1 tbsp. rice vinegar
pepper to taste

Preparation:
1. Toss ingredients together and serve.

How to Eat:
Eat a serving for lunch or dinner as a side dish.

Dinner Recipes

Bone Broth (Soup Stock)

When food becomes trendy it becomes intimidating. There is no need. Bone broth is just old fashioned soup stock. Bones and other inedible leftovers are cooked in water for hours. It was a process born of a desperate need for nutrition which resulted in superior taste and Jing tonification. Jing is concentrated in bone marrow and connective tissue of joints. Slow cooking for hours with a little vinegar extracts the Jing and delivers it in a highly digestible form. Vegetarians will also benefit from deeply extracting nutrients from vegetable-based broth. If this process is too laborious you can substitute store-bought soup stock.

Basic Rules of Broth:[39]

1. Rinse bones first and blanch to remove dirt and blood.
2. Roast bones in the oven for 1-2 hours greatly increases flavor.
3. Use a combination of long bones, tendons, feet, and odds and ends.
4. Leftover chicken or fish carcasses can be used.
5. Cook stock at low, continuous temperature.
6. Cook animal parts 6 or more hours. Add vegetables during the final 45 minutes of cooking.
7. At the end of cooking, gently strain the stock to make it transparent.

Begin with an approximate ratio:

- Bone broth: 1 lb. bones and bits : 1 qt. cold water : ½ cup vegetables
- Vegetable Broth: 1 cup vegetables : 1 qt. cold water

Postpartum Bone Broth

Comments:
This broth can be used in your soup recipes. Feel free to substitute ingredients you have on hand. Just be sure to keep the proportion on bones to vegetables.

Ingredients:
5 lbs. split bones with marrow, joints.
2 pork or beef trotters, have butcher split into pieces (pig's or cow's feet)
½ cup carrots, chopped
½ cup celery, chopped
½ cup beets, chopped
½ cup yam or winter squash, chopped

---

39. Adapted from Thomas Keller. *The French Laundry Cookbook.* (New York: Artisan, 1999).

½ cup mushrooms

1 large onion

2 cloves garlic (if no Heat signs)

packet Chinese herbs from TCM herbalist (optional)

2 tbsp. black rice, apple cider, or other vinegar

1 tsp. each: rosemary, thyme, clove

1 bunch fresh parsley, chopped

5 qt. cold water

Preparation:

1. Preheat oven to 425° F.
2. Bring pot of water to a boil. Rinse bones and trotters and place in boiling water for 5 minutes. Remove.
3. (Optional) Put bones (not trotters) in oven to roast for 1 hour until nicely browned.
4. Put bones and trotters in cold water over low heat. Skim bubbles and scum as they emerge from the surface. Once the water is clear add vinegar and rosemary, thyme, and clove.
5. After the broth has cooked for 4-5 hours add vegetables and herbs. Cook an additional 45 minutes. Add parsley and cook additional 5 minutes.
6. To strain, ladle slowly out of pot and through a fine colander. Take care not to agitate the broth. This is to avoid agitating the sediment at the bottom of the pot.

How to Use:

Once cooled, divide stock into airtight containers. Refrigerated stock will keep for a few days. The rest can be frozen.

Vegetable Broth

Comments:

This broth can be used in your soup recipes. Feel free to substitute ingredients you have on hand.

Ingredients:

3 carrots , chopped

3 stalks of celery, chopped

1 large onion, chopped[40]

2 medium beets, chopped

½ cup yam or winter squash, chopped

½ cup mushrooms, chopped

2 cloves garlic (if no Heat signs)

packet Chinese herbs from TCM herbalist (optional)

1 tsp each: rosemary, thyme, sage

---

40. The combination of celery, carrots, and onion is called "mirepoix" and is safe choice for use in all stocks and soups.

1 bay leaf
1 bunch fresh parsley, chopped
cold water to cover

Preparation:
1. Place ingredients (except for parsley) in a large saucepan and slowly bring to a simmer. Simmer for 45 minutes.
2. Add parsley and simmer additional 5 minutes. Strain.

How to Use:
Once cooled, divide stock into airtight containers. Refrigerated stock will keep for a few days. The rest can be frozen.

Quick Soup Stock

Comments:
If you have limited time, this makes a quick and flavorful broth.

Ingredients:
1 organic chicken or fish carcass
1 tomato, skin and seeds removed
1 carrot, chopped
1 onion, chopped
1 clove garlic, chopped
1tbsp. vinegar
1 bunch parsley, chopped
8 cups of water

Preparation:
1. Place ingredients in a large saucepan and bring to a boil. Simmer for 1 hour. Strain, conserving the broth, and discarding the rest.

How to Use:
Use as stock for soup, congee, or stew recipes.

Fish Soup Recipes

In traditional Taiwanese postpartum recovery, light, soft fish, such as Flathead Mullet fish (*Mugil cephalus*), Black Larvel, or Yellow Croaker fish (*Pseudosciaena crocea and polyactis*), is eaten for the first two weeks as it is easy to digest and helps build the strength of new mothers.[41] After two weeks richer fish is eaten.

Fish and Carrot Soup

Ingredients:
½ -1 lb. mild fish
lime to marinate fish
3 carrots, chopped
3 stalks celery, chopped
1 small onion, finely chopped
½ inch fresh ginger, finely chopped
1 bunch parsley or cilantro, chopped
black sesame oil to coat pan
2 cups soup stock
dash of rice wine

Preparation:
1. Rinse fish and marinate in lime juice for 10 minutes. Strain.
2. Coat medium saucepan with oil and place over medium-high heat. Add ginger and onion and sauté until browned but not blackened.
3. Add fish. Sear on both sides. Lower heat and allow to cook a few minutes. Be sure the fish is still soft when pressing down on it with a fork. Remove fish from heat and put aside.
4. Pour stock into saucepan and bring to a boil. Lower to a simmer. Add vegetables and cook 20 minutes. Add parsley or cilantro.
5. Add fish. Remove from heat and serve warm.

How to Eat:
Eat a bowl for dinner paired with sprouted grain toast.

Coconut Fish Soup

Comments:
Nourishes the body without causing congestion.

Ingredients:
½ pound of fish
1 tomato, chopped
1 carrot, finely chopped
½ cup broccoli, chopped

---

41. Shuqi Zhuang. *Postpartum Recovery Program; a Manual of Rules and Recipes for the Postpartum Woman.* (Taiwan: Guang He Chu Ban She, 2005). ISBN 9578807015

1 onion, finely chopped

1 lime, separate zest, and use for juice at the end

2 kaffir lime leaves, bruised

4 sprigs cilantro or parsley, chopped

½ inch ginger, grated

½ inch galangal, thinly sliced

½ cup coconut milk

1 ½ cups soup stock

1 tsp. black sesame oil

Preparation:

1. Bring stock to a boil. Reduce to a simmer. Add kaffir lime leaves, galangal, lime zest, carrot, broccoli, coconut milk, and chili peppers. Allow to simmer while preparing rest of ingredients.
2. Add black sesame oil to a frying pan over medium-high heat.
3. Add ginger and onions and sauté until browned.
4. Add fish. Sear on both sides. Lower heat and allow to cook a few minutes. Be sure the fish is still soft when pressing down on it with a fork.
5. Remove from heat and add to the soup stock. Add tomato, lime juice, and cilantro. Serve warm.

How to Eat:

Eat a bowl for dinner paired with sprouted grain toast.

Soups to Promote Lactation

Eating lactation-promoting soups three times a week promotes healthy breast milk production. Women should eat these soups as long as they continue to breast feed.

Carp and Tofu Soup

Comments:

Carp & Tofu Soup is a traditional recipe to increase healthy milk production. Carp is the preferred fish to promote lactation. It is also called grass carp or white amur (wan yú, 鯉魚). Recipes always include carp and tofu, but vary from that point. This is my version.

Ingredients:

1 carp tail

4 ounces extra firm tofu (non-GMO), cubed

¼ cup winter squash or pumpkin, cut into cubes

1 large tomato, diced

2 stalks celery, chopped

6 longan berries (*long yan rou*)

2 pieces astragalus (*huang qi*) or codonopsis root (*dang shen*) from a TCM herbalist (optional)

1 small onion, chopped

½ inch fresh ginger, grated

½ tsp. dill

1 lime

4 cups soup broth

dash of rice wine or dry sherry

black sesame seed or vegetable oil to coat pan

black sesame oil to coat pan

black or white pepper to taste

Preparation:
1. Place carp in a bowl and cover with lime juice for 15 minutes. Strain.
2. Coat a large saucepan with oil and place over medium-high heat. Add onions and ginger and sauté until browned. Add carp tail. Sauté on both sides until browned (about 5 minutes).
3. Add soup stock, tofu, squash, tomato, wine, dill, longan berries, yam, and celery to the pan. Bring to a boil, then reduce to a simmer. Cook for 45 minutes. Serve warm.

How to Eat:
Lactating mothers can eat a few times a week for dinner to promote abundant breast milk. In cases of scanty milk due to deficiency, eat 2 bowls a day, three days in a row.

Carp and Green Papaya Soup

Comments:
Carp and green papaya increase milk production.

Ingredients:
½ pound carp, washed and cut into pieces

1 cup green papaya, grated or cubed

5 red dates, pitted and chopped

½ inch piece fresh ginger, finely chopped

2 cups soup stock

black sesame oil to coat pan

white or black pepper to taste

Preparation:
1. Bring stock to a boil. Add papaya and dates. Allow to simmer while preparing rest of ingredients.

2. Coat a frying pan with black sesame oil and place over medium-high heat. Add ginger and sauté until browned.

3. Add fish. Sear on both sides. Lower heat and allow to cook a few min. Be sure the fish is still soft when pressing down on it with a fork. Remove from heat and add to the soup stock. Serve warm.

How to Eat:
Lactating mothers can eat a few times a week for dinner to promote abundant breast milk. In cases of scanty milk due to deficiency, eat 2 bowls a day, three days in a row.

BOOSTING LACTATION

These lactation recipes have been used for centuries to promote abundant, high quality breast milk while keeping the mother from getting depleted. Sometimes they surprise me at how well they work. I had a 37 year old patient who suffered from substantial Qi and Blood deficiency, with symptoms of frequent weepiness, pallor, low appetite, and fatigue. She looked fragile. She produced little breast milk and what came out was watery and thin. I recommended the Pork Trotter & Peanut Soup and gave her a packet of herbs to add. She did not like the idea of eating pork trotters so I suggested she strain everything out at the end and drink it like a tea. She took it for three days, twice a day and her breast milk production increased to a normal, healthy level. Even though she was satisfied with her breast milk, I was concerned that with her level of deficiency that she would soon become depleted again, I recommended that she take Qi and Blood tonic pills (which were more convenient for long-term use) and to make chicken soup three times a week for as long as she was breastfeeding. She continued to breast feed for about seven months, after which she had a plump, healthy baby and she felt recovered with a healthy glow to her.

Pork Trotter's & Peanut Soup

Comments:
Pork Trotter's & Peanut Soup is the quintessential lactation promoting recipe. This is my rendition of the traditional postpartum formula. It always contains pork trotters (or pig's feet) and peanuts, often with Chinese herbs. I find it tastes better to drink the herbs separately as a formula, but it is more effective therapeutically when taken together. This recipe not only promotes breast milk production. Its high collagen content makes it an excellent remedy to restore the pelvic floor, beautify the skin, and recover the joints.

Ingredients:
4 pork trotters (pig's feet), have butcher cut each one into 4 pieces
1 cup peanuts, raw and peeled
1 inch fresh ginger, chopped
2 carrots, chopped

3 stalks of celery, chopped

1 onion, chopped

½ cup shitake mushrooms or other mushrooms, stems removed

packet Chinese herbs in cheesecloth pouch from TCM herbalist (optional)

1 tbsp. vinegar

dash of rice wine, or other alcohol

water to cover

Seasoning:

1 tsp. each: rosemary, thyme, nutmeg

1 bay leaf

1 piece cinnamon bark

2 pieces of licorice root (*gan cao*) (optional)

1 clove garlic, minced (omit in Heat conditions)

1 piece dried orange peel (*chen pi*)

black or white pepper to taste

Preparation:

1. Bring big pot of water to a boil. Add pork trotters. Boil for 5 minutes. Remove and rinse the trotters. Discard water.
2. Add pork trotters, seasoning, vinegar, and cold water to cover to a large saucepan or crockpot. Slowly bring to a simmer and cook for 2-4 hours until pork trotters are soft.
3. Add peanuts, ginger, vegetables, herbs (if using), and rice wine. Simmer an additional 30-45 minutes.
4. Remove pork trotters. Remove gelatinous material from the bones and cut into pieces. Discard bones and tough connective tissue. Fish out cinnamon bark, bay leaf, and herbs and discard. Serve warm.

How to Eat:

Lactating mothers can eat 1 bowl a few times a week to promote abundant breast milk and strengthen their bodies. In cases of scanty milk due to deficiency, eat 1 small bowl twice a day for three days in a row. This soup can be eaten anytime for rejuvenation, skin beautification, or joint health.

Cantonese-style Pork Trotters Soup[42]

Comments:

This is the Cantonese version of the classic postpartum dish. It warms the body, tonifies Qi and Blood, and promotes lactation. This is a warming recipe and should be taken only in small amounts or else avoided in cases of Heat or excess.

---

42. Also known as Pork Trotters in Black Vinegar or Pickled Pork Trotter Soup, 猪脚醋. Adapted from Shu Han. (2011). *Pork Trotters with Vinegar.* Retrieved from www.mummyicancook.com/2011/01/pork-trotters-with-vinegar.html

Ingredients:
2 pork trotters (pig's feet), have butcher cut each one into 4 pieces
2 inch piece of ginger, sliced
500ml bottle of black rice vinegar
1 cup peanuts, raw and peeled
water to cover
¼ cup raw sugar (muscovado) (optional)
4 peeled hard-boiled eggs
black sesame oil to coat pan

Preparation:
1. Bring a big saucepan full of water to a boil. Add pork trotters and boil for 5 minutes. Strain trotters and discard water.
2. Coat a large saucepan with black sesame oil and place over medium-high heat. Add ginger and sauté until it begins to brown. Add pork trotters and sauté until they begin to brown.
3. Add vinegar, peanuts, sugar (if using) and water to cover. Bring to a boil then simmer for 2-4 hours, until trotters are soft.
4. Add peeled hard-boiled eggs for additional 10-20 min. Remove from heat and serve warm.

How to Eat:
Lactating moms can eat a few times a week to promote abundant breast milk and strengthen their bodies. In cases of scanty milk due to deficiency, eat 1 small bowl twice a day, for three days in a row. This soup can be eaten anytime for rejuvenation, skin beautification, or joint health.

Vegan Soup Recipes

Pregnancy, the postpartum period, breastfeeding, and during menses are the most challenging times to be vegan. The body requires extra nutrients to replenish the Blood and rebuild hormone levels. Even small amounts of animal product strongly replenish the Blood, particularly when cooked with Blood-building herbs.

Strict vegans can supplement their diet with extra protein during these periods. Incorporate soy products and protein powders into the diet. Dishes can be prepared with Chinese herbs to increase their tonifying qualities. Try to eating eggs during these periods as they are concentrated and easily digestible Qi and Blood tonics.

Raw food diets are not advisable during the postpartum month. To substitute for the warmth of animal products, emphasize warming, tonifying vegetables such as carrots, winter squash, and beets.

Vegan Qi and Blood-building foods: Red jujube date (*hong zao*), black jujube date (*da zao*), blackstrap molasses, spirulina and chlorophyll-rich foods, lotus seeds (*lian zi*), leafy greens, black sesame seeds (*hei zhi ma*), go ji berries (*gou qi zi*), longan berries (*long yan rou*), carrots, beets, black beans, and chestnuts.

Vegan Blood-moving foods: Shitake mushrooms, garlic, eggplant, black wood ear mushroom (*hei mu er*), and cabbage.

African Peanut Soup[43]

Comments:
The peanuts and yams promote milk production.

Ingredients:
1 small winter squash (butternut, acorn, etc.)
1 yam, peeled and chopped
1 russet potato, peeled and chopped
2 carrots, chopped
3 stalks celery, chopped
1 zucchini squash, chopped
1 cup chopped leafy greens (collard greens, kale, chard, etc.)
1 onion, chopped
½ inch piece of fresh ginger, grated
1tsp. vegetable oil (safflower, grapeseed, or coconut)
1 clove garlic
1 tsp. each: curry powder, turmeric
½ tsp. cumin powder
black or white pepper to taste
4 cups soup stock
½ cup organic, non-GMO crunchy peanut butter

Preparation:
1. Bake winter squash at 325° F until soft (30minutes – 1 hour). Peel, remove seeds, and chop.
2. Put oil in large sauce pan over medium-high heat. Add onions, ginger, and garlic. Sauté until browned.
3. Add all ingredients to pot except peanut butter. Bring to a boil and simmer for 45 minutes.
4. Remove soup from heat and put in a VitaMix or other blender until completely blended.
5. Pour back into pot and mix in peanut butter. Serve.

How to Eat:
Eat as main course with sprouted grain toast.

---

43. Based on my mom, Dr. Judith Andrews', recipe.

Black Bean Soup

Comments:
Black beans tonify the Liver and Kidneys, and nourish Qi and Blood.

Ingredients:
1 cup black beans
½ cup winter squash, yam, or sweet potato, chopped
1 cup collard greens, chopped
1 bunch parsley
3 red dates (*hong zao*), pitted and chopped
5 longan berries (*long yan rou*)
1 clove garlic, minced (omit if Heat signs)
½ onion, chopped
½ inch ginger, grated
1 bay leaf
1 tsp. turmeric
½ tsp. powdered cumin
1 tsp. thyme
black and white pepper
3-4 cups soup stock or water
black sesame, olive, safflower or other oil to coat pan
dash of rice wine

Preparation:
1. Soak beans overnight. Drain.
2. Put water, beans, squash, dates, longan berries, bay leaf, cumin, turmeric, and thyme in a saucepan and bring to a boil. Simmer 45 minutes or until beans are cooked through. (Alternately, use a pressure cooker to cook in 20 minutes).
3. Put oil in a frying pan over medium-high heat. Add ginger, garlic, and onion. Sauté until browned. Add greens, parsley, and rice wine. Sauté for 1 minute. Add pepper to taste.
4. Remove from heat and add to beans. Mix and serve.

How to Eat:
Eat as main course with sprouted grain toast or eat with Yi Ren Rice.

Adzuki Bean Stew

Comments:
Adzuki beans (*chi xiao dou*) drain water weight, move stagnant blood, and promote lactation.

Ingredients:
1 cup red adzuki beans (*chi xiao dou*)

½ cup winter squash, yam, or sweet potato, chopped

1 cup swiss chard, chopped

1 bunch parsley

3 red dates (hong zao), pitted and chopped

5 longan berries (long yan rou)

1 clove garlic, minced (omit if Heat signs)

½ onion, chopped

½ inch ginger, grated

1 bay leaf

1 tsp. each: thyme, coriander

black or white pepper

3-4 cups soup stock or water

black sesame, olive, safflower or other oil to coat pan

dash of rice wine

Preparation:

1. Soak beans overnight. Drain.
2. Put water, beans, squash, dates, longan berries, bay leaf, coriander, and thyme in a saucepan and bring to a boil. Simmer for 45 minutes or until beans are cooked through. (Alternately, use a pressure cooker to cook in 20 minutes).
3. Put oil in a frying pan over medium-high heat. Add ginger, garlic, and onion. Sauté until browned. Add greens, parsley, and rice wine. Sauté for 1 min. Add pepper to taste.
4. Remove from heat and add to beans. Mix and serve.

How to Eat:

Eat as main course with sprouted grain toast or eat with Yi Ren Rice.

THE 5 BEANS FOR BALANCE

Besides being an excellent source of protein and fiber, different-colored beans are used to balance out the five organ systems. Red adzuki beans (*chi xiao dou*) benefit the Heart organ system, drain edema, and are used extensively for postpartum women. They also strengthen the Spleen, reduce edema and weight gain, clear Dampness and Heat, treat leukorrhea and diarrhea, and move stagnant Blood. Soy beans and garbanzo beans are alternately used to harmonize the Spleen organ system. Lima beans benefit the Lung organ system and beautify the skin. Black beans strengthen the Kidney organ system and nourish Blood and Yin. Mung beans (*lu dou*) benefit the Liver organ system, clear toxins and heavy metals, and resolve Damp-Heat.

Date & Squash Soup

Comments:
This soup includes a combination of food herbs and vegetables that nourish Qi and Blood.

Ingredients:
½ cup winter squash, chopped
½ cup sweet potato, chopped
1 medium tomato, chopped
½ onion, chopped
½ inch piece of ginger, grated
3 red dates (hong zao), pitted and chopped
¼ cup go ji berries (go qi zi)
2 tsp. spirulina (optional)
black sesame, olive, safflower or other oil to coat pan
3 cups of soup stock
black or white pepper to taste
dash of rice wine

Procedure:
1. Rinse dates and go ji berries.
2. Put oil in sauce pan over medium-high heat. Add ginger and onions. Sauté until browned.
3. Add soup stock and rest of the ingredients (except for spirulina). Bring to a boil, then simmer for 30 minutes. Remove from heat. Mix in spirulina to serving bowl while soup is still hot.

How to Eat:
Eat as main course with sprouted grain toast or eat with Yi Ren Rice.

Lentil Barley Stew[44]

Comments:
Barley supports milk production. Lentils tonify the Kidneys and Jing, and are a good source of protein.

Ingredients:
½ cup brown lentils
½ cup barley
8 ounces mushrooms, chopped
3 stalks of celery, chopped
2 carrots, chopped

---

44. Adapted from Sarah. (2013). *Vegan Lentil Barley Stew*. Retrieved from www. makingthymeforhealth .com/2013/10/22/vegan-lentil-barley-stew

15 ounce can diced tomatoes with liquid

1 onion, finely chopped

½ inch fresh ginger, grated

1 garlic clove, minced (optional, if no Heat signs)

½ cup rice wine or dry sherry

2 bay leaves

½ tsp. each: thyme, tarragon

5 cups vegetable broth

safflower, olive, or coconut oil to coat the pan

Preparation:
1. Rinse lentils and barley and soak overnight.
2. Coat a large saucepan with oil and place over medium-high heat. Add onions, then ginger and garlic. Sauté until browned.
3. Add carrots, celery, mushrooms, thyme, and tarragon. Sauté until they get some color. Add rice wine and simmer 10 minutes uncovered, allowing wine to reduce.
4. Add broth, tomatoes, bay leaves, barley, and lentils. Bring to a boil then reduce heat to a simmer. Cook for 45 minutes. Serve warm.

How to Eat:
Eat a serving for breakfast, lunch, or dinner.

Pumpkin Stew[45]

Comments:
This hearty, warming soup strengthens Qi and builds Blood. Garbanzo beans are high in iron and nourish the Spleen.

Ingredients:
1 small cooking pumpkin (sugar pumpkin, can substitute butternut squash), cubed

3 large potatoes, cubed

3 parsnips, chopped

8 ounce can garbanzo beans, drained

8 ounce frozen spinach, chopped and thawed

1 tbsp. go ji berries (*gou qi zi*)

2 medium onions, chopped

½ inch fresh ginger, grated

1 cinnamon stick

1 tsp. coriander

½ tsp. cumin

---

45. Inspired by Santopietro, Jill. (2011). *Slow Cooker Root Vegetable Stew.* Retrieved from www.chow.com/recipes/29347-slow-cooker-root-vegetable-stew

3 cups soup broth

1 tbsp. apple cider or rice vinegar

olive, safflower, or coconut oil to coat pan

Preparation:

1. Coat a large frying pan with oil and place over medium-high heat. Add onions, then ginger. Sauté until browned. Add cinnamon stick, coriander, and cumin and sauté until fragrant.
2. Transfer to a slow cooker. Add pumpkin, potatoes, parsnips, garbanzo beans, spinach, broth, and vinegar. Set to high and cook 2-3 hours.
3. Remove from heat and serve warm.

How to Eat:

Eat a serving for lunch or dinner.

THE POWER OF ORANGE

Orange vegetables are very helpful for postpartum women. Yam and sweet potato strengthen digestion (Spleen and Stomach Qi), are laxative, and increase Yin fluids. They alleviate postpartum constipation, visual weakness, and insufficient lactation. Pumpkin strengthens digestion (Spleen and Stomach Qi) and transforms Phlegm-Damp. It helps stabilize the fetus during pregnancy (protects against miscarriage) and treats diabetes.

Probiotics & Digestives

The combination of Qi deficiency, antibiotics and anesthesia used during birth, and inactivity can lead to gas, constipation, and digestive upset. Postpartum women should take probiotics daily. These can be taken as a supplement or simply eat probiotic foods twice daily with meals. Probiotic foods include kefir, sauerkraut, kimchi, yogurt, natural pickles, and kombucha tea. Of these, kefir is the simplest to make yourself and can be made from milk or by using sugar water or juice. Postpartum women should also take digestive remedies with meals. Plain green, oolong, or pu-erh tea help digest fats, but should not be taken with supplements.

Milk Kefir

Comments:
Milk kefir populates the digestive tract will beneficial bacteria, providing probiotics and digestive enzymes. Cow's milk or goat's milk can be used. Goat's milk is a Yang tonic, with a warming thermal property, and better tolerated by some. Low fat or full fat milk can be used, however, the milk must be organic and as natural as possible. Kefir grains are an excellent indicator of the quality of milk, as they don't proliferate in the presence of antibiotics and chemicals. Do not let metal utensils come in contact with kefir grains. Use plastic or wooden spoons and a plastic strainer. Note: Kefir grains proliferate after repeated fermentations so you will want to share them with others.

Ingredients:
1½ cups organic milk
1 tbsp. kefir grains

Preparation:
1. Place ingredients in a glass. Cover with paper towel or cheesecloth and a rubber band.
2. Let sit 12-24 hours. Less time is required in warmer temperatures, more in colder.
3. Strain with a plastic colander. Place grains in new milk. Drink the strained kefir milk.

A POWERFUL PROBIOTIC

Milk kefir can correct digestive upset even under extreme conditions. One of my patients got a serious bacterial infection and was on IV antibiotics for two weeks. Within days of starting treatment he developed thrush; a thick white fur coated his tongue, which signaled yeast overgrowth, Dampness, and Spleen weakness. He also suffered from low appetite and lethargy. He was prohibited from taking any herbs or supplements so I recommended he try plain milk kefir. Even though milk kefir is dairy-based, which usually exacerbates Dampness, it resolved the tongue coating and aversion to food within 2 days. He would eat about ¼ - ½ a cup twice a day. After the first time he took it he craved it plain, with no spices or sweeteners.

How to Drink:

Use kefir milk in small doses throughout the day. Dairy is cooling and moistening. Add a little pungent spice such as pepper, cardamom, ginger, nutmeg, or coriander to balance. Kefir grains can be stored in milk in the refrigerator up to one week. If not used regularly, it can be dehydrated and frozen for long-term storage.

Water Kefir

Comments:

To reduce dairy intake, you can opt to drink water kefir. Water kefir grains are a different microorganism but the process is similar. You can use coconut water, raw sugar water, or diluted apple juice instead of milk. Established milk kefir grains can be adapted to use with coconut water. microorganism.

Ingredients:

1½ cups water + 1 tbsp. raw sugar (muscovado) (or 1 ½ cups coconut water, or ½ cup organic apple juice + 1 cup water)
1 tbsp. water kefir grains

Preparation:

1. Place ingredients in a glass. Cover with paper towel or cheesecloth and a rubber band.
2. Let sit 12-24 hours. Less time is required in warmer temperatures, more in colder.
3. Strain with plastic colander. Place grains in new sugar water or coconut water. Drink the strained kefir water.

How to Drink:

Drink ¼ cup of kefir water with or between meals.

Longan & Go Ji Kefir

Comments:

You can make kefir water more interesting and nutritious by flavoring it with fruits and spices. Note: be sure to strain out kefir grains first or they may be injured by the additives.

Ingredients:

1½ cups kefir water
1 tbsp. go ji berries (*gou qi zi*)
3 longan berries (*long yan rou*)

Preparation:

1. Place ingredients in a glass. Cover with paper towel or cheesecloth and a rubber band.
2. Let sit 12-24 hours. Less time is required in warmer temperatures, more in colder.
3. Strain with plastic colander. Discard the berries. Drink the strained kefir water.

How to Drink:
Drink ¼ cup of kefir water with or between meals.

Ume Plum Tea

Comments:
Ume plum[46] is a Japanese fruit reminiscent of a sour apricot. Umeboshi is ume plum that has been pickled with any of a variety of ingredients including bonito flakes, kombu, or honey. For digestive health purposes choose umeboshi plum made with red shiso leaves (perilla leaf, *zi su ye*), a heavy dose of salt, and shochu, a Japanese alcohol. This is the most common form seen in American health food stores. They should be reddish brown, and free of MSG, sugar, and artificial dyes. Umeboshi is anti-parasitic and promotes digestion. Vinegar in general stimulates the Liver, disperses Qi and Blood stagnation, and improves digestion. Vinegar and fermented foods compensate for low stomach acids and enzymes to break down foods.[47] Tea aids digestion and rids the body of fats.

Ingredients:
1 umeboshi plum
½ tsp tea (green, pu-erh, or oolong)
hot water

Preparation:
1. Bring water to a boil.
2. Mash umeboshi plum in a mug (be careful of the pit).
3. Add hot water. Place a teabag or loose tea in a teaball in the mug to steep.
4. Allow to steep for 3-5 minutes. Remove tea and ume pit. Drink tea warm with pieces of ume.

How to Drink:
Drink with meals.

Green Tea & Hawthorn Berry

Comments:
Hawthorn berry (*shan zha*) is particularly helpful to digest protein, however it is very acid and can aggravate acid reflux in some. Drink this recipe in lieu of Hawthorn Berry Tea (page 161) if there is also digestive weakness. Tea aids digestion and rids the body of fats. Dried tangerine peel (*chen pi*) promotes healthy water metabolism and reduces Phlegm.

---

46. TCM uses smoked ume plums, known as *wu mei*. The smoked version treats diarrhea and parasites.
47. Taking 1 tsp. of apple cider vinegar with meals can help treat high blood sugar in some individuals. Be careful in cases of acid reflux, and avoid contact of vinegar with teeth to avoid damage to enamel. I recommend using a straw when drinking vinegar or lemon juice in water.

Ingredients:
1 tsp green, oolong, or pu-erh tea
1 tbsp. hawthorn berries (*shan zha*)
1 tbsp. dried tangerine peel (*chen pi*)
raw sugar (muscovado), or other sweetener to taste
2½ cups water

Preparation:
1. Rinse ingredients and place in a medium saucepan or kettle with water. Bring to a boil and simmer 10 minutes.
2. Strain and serve warm.

How to Drink:
Drink with meals.

Daikon Radish Slices

Comments:
Daikon radish dissolves Phlegm, clears Heat, and promotes digestion.

Ingredients:
raw daikon radish

Preparation:
1. Cut 2-3 thin slices of daikon.

How to Eat:
Eat with meals.

Dessert Recipes

Sugary desserts are not health-promoting and should be kept to a minimum. Instead eat fruit or nutrient dense desserts such as the recipes below.

Sweet Adzuki Bean Soup

Comments:
This is the same recipe as Adzuki Bean Tea, but with less water. It is common in Asian cooking to eat adzuki beans (chi xiao dou) in desserts or as sweet soup.

Ingredients:
1 cup red adzuki beans (chi xiao dou)
2 cups water
1 bay leaf
1 tsp. coriander
1 inch fresh ginger, chopped
raw sugar (muscovado), or other sweetener to taste
dash of rice wine (optional)

Procedure:
1. Soak beans 8 hours or overnight.
2. Place beans and water in saucepan. Bring to a boil and skim off bubbles.
3. Add bay leaf, coriander, and ginger. Add dash of rice wine (optional). Simmer for 1 hour or until beans are thoroughly cooked.
4. Add sweetener (optional) and serve.

How to Eat:
Eat a small bowl as a dessert or snack.

8 Treasure Rice

Comments:
This is a traditional tonifying dish providing a powerhouse of superfoods. The 8 herbs vary according to the recipe. White sweet rice is generally used. This recipe uses black sweet rice, as it is more tonifying for the Blood and Kidneys. The recipe is traditionally steamed. I use a rice cooker as it is the easiest method though it doesn't look as pretty as when it is steamed. Sweet rice does not cook well in a regular saucepan and sticks to the pot. Replace some of the water with coconut milk to transform it into a rich dessert.

Ingredients:
5. 1 cup black glutinous (sweet) rice

6 lotus nuts (*lian zi*)

6 longan berries (*long yan rou*)

¼ cup go ji berries (*gou ji zi*)

¼ cup black sesame seeds (*hei zhi ma*)

1 tbsp. tangerine peel (*chen pi*), crushed

4 pieces poria (*fu ling*), crushed

6 red dates (*hong zao*), pitted and chopped

¼ cup adzuki beans (*chi xiao dou*)

raw sugar (muscovado), or other sweetener to taste

2½ cups water (or as directed on rice cooker, or can substitute some water with coconut milk)

Preparation:

1. Rinse rice and beans and soak 8 hours or overnight. Drain
2. Place ingredients in rice cooker and cook.

How to Eat:

Eat with meals, as snack, or as dessert.

Raw Go Ji Lime Truffles

Comments:

Everyone needs a treat now and again. These are an easy, yet decadent, dessert based on a delicious macaroon recipe.[48] Be sure to make small portions and eat sparingly. This recipe tonifies Blood and Yin.

Ingredients:

1½ cups almond flour

1½ cups dried shredded unsweetened coconut

¼ cup go ji berries (*gou qi zi*)

pinch of salt

6 tbsp. raw honey (or agave or Grade B maple syrup)

6 tbsp. lime or lemon juice

2 tsp. vanilla

zest from 1 lime or lemon

¼ cup + 1 tbsp. melted coconut oil

Preparation:

1. Mix together dry ingredients in a medium-sized bowl: almond flour, shredded coconut, go ji berries, and salt. Set aside.
2. In a mixer, combine honey, lime juice, vanilla, and lemon zest.

---

48. Adapted from Yvonne. (2013). *Coco-roons.* Retrieved from www.triedandtasty.com/2013/07/coco-roons

3. Slowly add dry ingredients to wet ingredients. Once combined, while your mixer is on, slowly pour in the melted coconut oil. Batter will thicken fairly quickly.
4. Use a 1 inch cookie scoop to form in to balls. Place on a cookie sheet and refrigerate for at least an hour.

How to Eat:
Eat 1 or 2 as a snack or dessert.

Raw Cacao Truffles

Comments:
This is the chocolate version. Be sure to make small portions and eat sparingly.

Ingredients:
1½ cups almond flour
1½ cups dried shredded unsweetened coconut
pinch of salt
6 tbsp. raw honey (or agave or Grade B maple syrup)
6 tbsp. coffee
2 tsp. vanilla
2 tbsp. raw cacao powder
¼ cup + 1 tbsp. melted coconut oil

Preparation:
1. Mix together dry ingredients in a medium-sized bowl: almond flour, shredded coconut, cacao, and salt. Set aside.
2. In a mixer, combine the honey, coffee, and vanilla.
3. Slowly add dry ingredients to wet ingredients. Once combined, while your mixer is on, slowly pour in the melted coconut oil.
4. Use a 1 inch cookie scoop to form in to balls. Place on a cookie sheet and refrigerate for at least an hour.

How to Eat:
Eat 1 or 2 as a snack or dessert.

Black Sesame Truffles

Comments:
Walnuts and black sesame seeds (*hei zhi ma*) tonify the Kidneys, nourish Jing, beautify the hair, and promote lactation. Raw honey balances and detoxifies the Liver, treats constipation, and drains Phlegm-Damp. Polygonatum root (*he shou wu*) is a longevity tonic that nourishes Blood.

Ingredients:

1 cup walnut (*hu tao ren*) meal

1 cup black sesame seed (*hei zhi ma*) meal

1 tbsp. ground polygonatum root (*he shou wu*) from TCM herbalist (optional)

6 tbsp. raw honey

¼ cup + 1 tbsp. melted coconut oil

Preparation:

1. To make the meal simply place walnuts and black sesame seeds in a blender to powder.
2. Combine walnut, black sesame seed, (polygonatum root powder if using), and honey in bowl and mix with a mixer until thoroughly blended.
3. Once combined, while your mixer is on, slowly pour in the melted coconut oil. Use a 1 inch cookie scoop to form in to balls. Place on a cookie sheet and refrigerate for at least an hour.

How to Eat:

Eat 1 or 2 as a snack or dessert.

Go Ji Pumpkin Cake

Comments:

This is a dairy and gluten-free, low sugar recipe to satisfy your sweet tooth. Pumpkin tonifies Qi and Yin. Molasses tonify Blood. Walnuts (hu tao ren) and go ji berries (*go qi zi*) tonify Kidney Jing. You can substitute boiled and mashed yam or sweet potato for the pumpkin.

Ingredients:

1¾ cups oat flour[49]

8-ounce can pumpkin (1 cup)

1 cup applesauce

1 tbsp. go ji berries (*gou qi zi*)

2 tsp. baking soda

1 tsp. baking powder

1 tsp. each: cinnamon, nutmeg, salt

½ tsp. allspice

¼ tsp. each: cloves, ginger powder

1 tsp. vanilla extract

¼ cup melted coconut oil, safflower, or other vegetable oil

1/3 cup raw honey

¼ cup molasses

---

49. Oat flour is moistening and ideal of dryness, Yin deficiency, and Blood deficiency. If there is gluten-intolerance or Phlegm-Damp (sinus congestion, edema, no desire to drink, abdominal bloating, vaginal discharge, mucous in stools) replace oat flour with a more drying option such as toasted buckwheat (kasha) flour. You can buy kasha and powder it in a blender such as a Vita-Mix.

¼ cup walnuts

1/3 cup water

Preparation:

1. Preheat oven to 350° F. Grease and flour a 9 by 10 inch loaf pan and set aside.
2. In a large bowl, mix together the dry ingredients. In another separate bowl, slowly combine the pumpkin, applesauce, coconut oil, honey, molasses and water.
3. Add the wet ingredients to the dry and fold until combined. Pour batter into the 9 by 10 inch prepared loaf pan. Bake for one hour or until a toothpick inserted in the middle comes out clean.

How to Eat:

Cut into squares and eat 1 or 2 as a snack or dessert.

Mung Bean & Seaweed Soup

Comments:

This is a traditional summer dessert in Vietnam and other parts of southeast Asia. Mung beans clear Heat, Toxic Heat, and resolve Dampness. Kombu seaweed dissolves Phlegm and masses of all kinds, and drains edema. Together they treat a wide variety of conditions such as acne, water retention, muscle inflammation, heat stroke, toxic exposure, and growths. This is a detoxifying recipe, however, if a postpartum woman is running hot, or if the weather is very warm and humid, this recipe is ideal. Cooking cool-natured foods, like in this recipe, is gentler on her system than it would be to incorporate raw vegetables or dairy into the diet. It is also an excellent dessert if you are concerned about Phlegm-Damp or losing weight. The sweet taste is balanced with bitter, bland, and salty tastes, making it deceptively more cleansing than tonifying.

Ingredients:

½ cup mung beans (*lu dou*)

2” x 5” piece of kombu seaweed (kelp, *kun bu*)

raw sugar (muscovado), xylitol, stevia, or other sweetener to taste

2 cups water

Preparation:

1. Rinse mung beans. Soak overnight. Strain.
2. Rinse kombu seaweed and add to a medium saucepan with mung beans and water.
3. Bring to a boil and simmer covered for 45 minutes, adding more water as necessary.
4. Remove from heat and add sweetener as desired.

How to Eat:

Have a bowl as a snack or dessert.

A SNEAKY WAY TO HIDE SEAWEED

My mom, Dr. Judith Andrews, does not care for seaweed and can usually sniff it out of a recipe. She surprised me when she really liked Mung Bean Seaweed Soup. The combination of mung bean and seaweed somehow takes the "sea" flavor into another direction. It is similar to how honeydew melon balances bitter melon.[1] Note: if you are serving it to someone who does not like seaweed, be sure to remove the seaweed before they see it.

[1]See "Bitter Melon Juice" recipe in Lia Andrews. *7 Times a Woman; Ancient Wisdom on Health & Beauty for Every Stage of Your Life*. (San Diego: Alcyone Press, 2013).

Appendices

Appendix A - Table of Chinese Herbs

English Common Name	Pin Yin	Botanical Name	Pharmaceutical Name	Chinese Characters
artemesia argyi, mugwort	Ài Yè	*Artemesia argyi*	Folium Artemesiae Argyi	艾叶
American ginseng	Xī Yáng Shēn	*Panax quinqueflium*	Radix Panacis Quinquefolii	西洋参
amomum	Shā Rén	*Amomum villosum*	Fructus Amomi	砂仁
barley sprouts, malt	Mài Yá	*Hordeum vulgare*	Fructus Hordei Germinatus	麦芽
bitter nail tea	Kŭ Dīng Chá	*Ligustrum robustum (loose leaf) or Ilex kudingcha(in nails)*		苦丁茶
black jujube, date	Dà Zăo	*Ziziphus jujuba*	Fructus Jujubae	大枣
black sesame seed	Hēi Zhī Ma	*Sesamum indicum L.*	Semen Sesami Nigrum	黑芝麻
black wood ear fungus	Hēi Mù Ěr		Auricularia Auricula Fungus	黑木耳
Chinese yam, dioscorea	(Huai) Shān Yào	*Dioscorea opposita*	Rhizoma Dioscoreae	山药
chrysanthemum flower	Jú Huā	*Chrysanthemum morifolium*	Flos Chrysanthemi	菊花
cinnamon bark	Ròu Guì	*Cinnamomum cassia*	Cortex Cinnamomi	肉桂
coix seed, Job's tears	Yì Yǐ Rén	*Coix lacryma-jobi*	Semen Coicis	薏苡仁
corn silk	Yù Mǐ Xū	*Zea mays*	Stigma Maydis	玉米须
deer antler	Lù Róng	*Cervus nippon*	Cornu Cervi Pantotrichum	鹿茸
deer horn (sliced)	Lù Jiăo (Pian)	*Cervus nippon*	Cornu Cervi	鹿角
dodder seed, cuscuta	Tù Sī Zĭ	*Cuscuta chinensis*	Semen Cuscutae	菟丝子
dolichos nut	Bái Biăn Dòu	*Dolichos lalab*	Semen Lablab Album	白扁豆
eucommia bark	Dù Zhòng	*Eucommia ulmoides*	Cortex Eucommiae	杜仲
fox nut, gorgon fruit	Qiàn Shí	*Euryale ferox*	Semen Euryales	芡實

ginger (fresh)	Shēng Jiāng	*Zinziber officinale*	Rhizoma Zingiberis Recens	生姜
ginseng	Rén Shēn	*Panax ginseng*	Radix Ginseng	人参
gou ji berries	Gōu Qǐ Zǐ	*Lycium barbarum L.*	Fructus Lycii	枸杞子
guan yin, clerodendri	Guān Yīn Chuàn	*Clerodendron Cyrtophyllum*	Radix cum Stem Clerodendri	觀音串
hawthorn berry	Shān Zhā	*Crataegus cuneata*	Fructus Crataegi	山楂
hemp seed, cannabis seed	Huǒ Má Rén	*Cannabis sativa*	Cannabis Semen	火麻仁
kelp	Kūn Bù	*Laminaria japonica*	Eckloniae Thallus	昆布
licorice root	Gān Cǎo	*Glycyrrhiza uralensis*	Radix Glycyrrhizae	甘草
lithospermum root	Zǐ Cǎo (Gēn)	*Lithospermum erythrorhizon*	Radix Lithospermi	紫草 (根)
longan fruit	Long Yǎn Ròu	*Euphoria longan*	Arillus Longan	龙眼肉
lotus nut	Lián Zǐ	*Nelumbo nucifera*	Semen Nelumbinis	莲子
lychee shell	Lì Zhī Ké (Qiào)	*Litchi chinensis*	Pericarpium Litchi	荔枝殼
mint	Bò He	*Mentha haplocalyx*	Herba Menthae	薄荷
motherwort	Yì Mǔ Cǎo	*Leonurus heterophyllus*	Herba Leonuri	益母草
mulberries	Sāng Shèn Zǐ	*Morus alba L.*	Fructus Mori	桑椹子
papaya	Mù Guā	*Chaenomeles lagenaria*	Fructus Chaenomelis	木瓜
placenta	Zǐ Hé Chē	*Homo sapiens*	Placenta Hominis	紫河车
poria	Fú Líng	*Poria cocos*	Poria	茯苓
Pseudoginseng, notoginseng	Sān Qī	*Panax notoginseng*	Radix Notoginseng	三七
red adzuki bean	Chì Xiǎo Dòu	*Phaseolus calcaratus*	Semen Phaseoli	赤小豆
red ginseng, steamed ginseng root (Korean or Chinese)	Hóng Shēn	*Panax ginseng*	Radix Ginseng	红参
red jujube, date	Hóng Zǎo	*Ziziphus jujuba*	Fructus Jujubae	红枣
reishi mushroom, ganoderma	Líng Zhī	*Ganoderma lucidum*	Ganoderma	靈芝
rose flower	Méi Gui Huā			玫瑰花

schizandra berry, Chinese magnolia vine fruit	Wǔ Wèi Zi	*Schisandra chinensis*	Fructus Schisandrae Chinensis	五味子
tangerine peel	Chén Pí	*Citrus reticulata*	Pericarpium Citri Reticulatae	陈皮
walnut	Hú Táo Rén	*Juglans regia*	Semen Juglandis	胡桃仁
white atractylodes	Bái Zhú	*Atractylodes macrocephala*	Rhizoma Atractylodis Macrocephalae	白朮
white cloud mushroom or fungus, white wood ear	Bái Mù Ěr	*Tremella fuciformis*	Fructificatio Tremellae Fuciformis	白木耳, 雪耳

Appendix B - Glossary of Terminology

5 Elements (五行, wǔxíng) – The 5 Elements are Wood, Fire, Earth, Metal, and Water. During the creation of the universe, there was a split between Yin and Yang. This polarity gave birth to the 5 Elements, also known as the 5 Phases. The 5 Elements can be used to describe interaction on all levels of existence, such as between the organs within the body, aspects of the psyche, interactions between people, and seasonal changes.

Acupuncture (针砭, zhēnbiān, or 针刺, zhēncì) – Refers to inserting tiny needles into specific points in the body called acupuncture points. Acupuncture points are places where energy pools along energy pathways.

(Western) Allopathic Medicine – What is typically referred to as standard or conventional Western medicine. It refers to biomedical interventions, such as pharmaceuticals and surgery, to combat disease. Allopathic medicine defines itself as being evidence-based and distinct from "alternative therapies," though there is mounting scientific evidence for alternative therapies as well. This term is controversial in some circles as it was originally used to distinguish it from homeopathy. It is not intended as a pejorative, rather it is used for lack of a better term to differentiate it from other forms of Western medicine such as osteopathy, naturopathy, and homeopathy.

Blood (血, xuè) – In Traditional Chinese Medicine contains the Qi and houses the Spirit. Blood is the physical manifestation of Qi and is inseparable from it. Qi gives life to the Blood, while Blood gives Qi physical form. Blood is moistening and lubricates the sinews and tendons and nourishes the skin and hair.

Blood Deficiency (血虚, xuèxū) – Lack of Blood refers to a lack of substance, as Blood lubricates the body and houses the Mind and Spirit. Common symptoms are pallor, dry skin, emotional and physical sensitivity, insomnia, blurred vision, timidity, pale and light menstrual bleeding with long cycles. Blood deficiency can be due to constitution or caused by blood loss, digestive weakness, poor eating and lifestyle, overwork (especially on the computer), excessive caretaking, and emotional trauma or loss. Affects the Heart and Liver. Blood deficiency is characterized by a pale, thin tongue and thin pulse.

Blood Stagnation (血淤, xuèyū) – Typical symptoms include stabbing, intense, fixed pain. Anything purple, visible dark veins, or blood clots indicates Blood Stagnation. Blood stagnation occurs due to physical or emotional trauma, longstanding Qi stagnation, or Cold invasion. Emotionally it can present as severe depression or insomnia years after physical or emotional trauma. Blood stagnation produces a purple tongue body or dark sublingual veins and a wiry or choppy pulse.

Cold (寒, hán) – It can either be due to external invasion or due to an internal deficiency of Qi or Yang. Cold is causes constriction and chills and is alleviated by warmth. The tongue will be pale or have a white coating and the pulse will be slow or tight.

Constitution – Refers to the strengths and weaknesses of the body. This is largely influenced by the Jing inherited from the parents and care during infancy and early childhood. Diet and lifestyle continuously influence the constitution. The constitution is slow to change. Understanding the constitution gives the ability to predict the outcome of disease and dictates lifestyle and diet choices.

Dampness (湿气, shīqì) – The terms Phlegm and Dampness refer to the congestion of body fluids in different manifestations. Dampness refers to the Middle and Lower Jiaos where it manifests as mucus and bloating in the digestive tract, copious white vaginal discharge, or cloudy and dribbling urination. Dampness can get lodged in the joints causing joint pain or under the skin causing edema and excess weight. Dampness shows itself on the tongue as a thick, greasy coating and as a slippery pulse.

Damp-Heat (濕熱, shīrè) – Refers to a combination of Dampness and Heat. It is most often a complication of longstanding digestive issues, Heat, or stagnation. Damp-Heat manifests as an inability to digest fats, abdominal bloating, yellow vaginal discharge, anger, resentment, indecisiveness, thirst with inability to drink, and red, itchy, and weepy skin conditions. It affects the Liver, Gallbladder, Urinary Bladder, Lower Jiao, and Large Intestine organ systems. It presents as a red tongue with yellow coating and slippery, rapid pulse.

Food Stagnation (家食, jiāshí) – Occurs when more food is ingested than the digestive system can process; either because food consumption is excessive or inappropriate or digestion is weak. Symptoms include belching, bad breath, abdominal bloating, lack of appetite, foul smelling stools, and insomnia. The tongue will have a thick white or yellow coating and the pulse will be slippery.

Heat (热, rè) – Causes inflammation, redness, agitation, bitter taste in the mouth, sensation of heat, excessive hunger, halitosis, or strong body odor. Symptoms are alleviated by cold. Heat can be due to external invasion, in the form of a pathogen (such as bacterial infection) or internally generated due to Yin deficiency, longstanding stagnation, or constitution. Heat creates a red tongue body or yellow tongue coating and rapid or full pulse.

Hun (Ethereal soul) (魂, hún) – The spirit of the Liver. The Hun is the Yang aspect of the soul; the part of the soul that moves and is insubstantial. The Hun connects the individual to the collective, is responsible for dreams, and is connected to creativity. In cases of Liver Blood deficiency, the Hun is not anchored, leading to insomnia and daydreaming.

Inner Alchemy (內丹, nèidān) – Refers to Daoist doctrines and practices designed to refine the inner landscape by transmuting negative thoughts, bad habits, sabotaging emotions, and other impediments to spiritual growth and physical vitality. There are many schools of Inner Alchemy passed down through various lineages.

Jade Egg (玉蛋, yùdàn) – A traditional tool to develop the vaginal muscles in Inner Alchemy exercises. Traditionally jade was formed into "eggs" and placed inside the vaginal canal. Jade increases Yin and seemed like the appropriate stone for this purpose. Currently eggs are available in a variety of stones.

Jade Gate (玉门, yùmén) – A metaphor for the vulva and vaginal canal.

Jing (Essence) (精, jīng) – The product of what is inherited from the parents and what is taken in from the environment (through eating and breathing). It is stored in the Kidneys but also circulates throughout the body. It is influenced by diet, lifestyle, and herbs. It relates to the individual's constitution which is possible, yet difficult to alter. Kidney Jing guides our maturation, development, and reproduction. It is the slow, fluid movement of the Kidney Jing that is described in the 7 year cycles women experience.

Jing Deficiency (精虚, jīng xū) – is a combination of Yin and Yang deficiency presenting with weak teeth, softening of bones, low back soreness, and hair loss. The natural decline of Jing with age signals the beginning of menopause. In younger people can present as developmental abnormalities, infertility, or constitutional weaknesses. Jing deficiency can be constitutional or due to aging, overwork, or excessive drug use, particularly methamphetamines. The tongue will vary depending if Yin or Yang is weaker and the pulse will be deep and weak.

Meridians (经线, jīngxiàn) – The pathways or circuits of energy flow through the body, also called Channels.

Moxibustion (moxa) (艾炷灸, àizhùjiǔ) – A central therapy in Traditional Chinese Medicine, often used with acupuncture during treatment. The leaves of Ai Ye (mugwort) are dried then formed into cones, sticks, or left loose, after which it is called "moxa." Moxa can be burned directly or indirectly on acupuncture points to warm the meridians and stimulate the flow of Qi.

Phlegm (痰, tán) – The terms Phlegm and Dampness refer to the congestion of body fluids in different manifestations. Phlegm can affect the Upper Jiao (Lungs, nose) causing symptoms such as excess mucus in the lungs, runny nose, and sinus congestion. It can present as Insubstantial Phlegm (also called Invsible or Dry Phlegm) where there may not be visible signs of excess mucus, but rather presents as mental impairment causing foggy thinking, poor cognition, manic depression, and irrational behavior. Phlegm can also manifest in certain channel pathology where there is paralysis and severe obstruction of the channels. Many modern diseases have a component of Phlegm such as high cholesterol and tumor formation. Phlegm produces an enlarged tongue body and a slippery pulse.

Po (Corporeal soul) (魄, pò) – The spirit of the Lungs. The Po is the Yin aspect of the soul; the part of the soul that guides the creation of the physical body. The Po defines the individual as separate, is responsible for instinct, is connected the physical senses. Imbalance in the Lungs and Large Intestine can cause dysfunction in proper boundaries.

Qi (气, qì) – Literally translates as "life force energy" or "vital energy." It is insubstantial. Qi can be felt (and seen by some), but it does not have form. It is what enlivens the body; like electricity that lights up a house. Qi has six functions within the body: transforming, transporting, holding, raising, protecting, and warming.

Qi Deficiency (气虚, qìxū) – Weakness of Qi causes weakness of function with symptoms like fatigue, weak limbs, poor muscle tone, bloating, craving for sweets, low immunity, pale menstrual blood and short menstrual cycles. It can be constitutional or caused by poor eating and sleeping habits, overwork, and stress. Qi deficiency can affect the Spleen, Lung, Heart, and Kidney organ systems. Qi deficiency is characterized by a pale tongue and weak pulse.

Qi Stagnation (气滞, qìzhì) – When Qi flow is impeded or stuck it causes symptoms like depression, stiffness, irritability, irregularity of mood, bowel movement, or menstrual cycles, fatigue, and frequent sighing. Qi stagnation involves the Liver organ system or the local area. It is most often caused by emotional stress or toxins, or local trauma. It can also be due to Qi deficiency.

Qigong (气功, qìgōng) – Qigong literally translates as "Qi exercise." It uses meditation, movement, and breath for healing and optimizing health. There are many styles of qigong. Qigong heals the physical, emotional, and spiritual bodies and can be used for self-healing or healing others.

Rice Wine (米酒, mǐjiǔ or 黄酒, huángjiǔ)– Chinese rice wine is similar to sake in that it is made from rice and kōji (曲霉菌, qū méi jūn, Aspergillus oryzae, a mold that breaks down rice starch into available sugars). However, it is processed and aged like wine, and may have a variety of other molds and yeasts added to it during fermentation such as red rice yeast (红曲米, hóng qū mǐ, Monascus purpureus). Chinese rice wine varies in color from yellow to brown, has a 17-20% alcohol content, and tastes similar to dry sherry. Look for drinking wines and avoid the lower grade cooking wines. Shaoxing rice wine (绍兴酒) is a popular wine made with red rice yeast that can be found inexpensively at Asian markets. Huadiao jiu (花雕酒), or nu'er hong (女儿红), is another popular style of rice wine made of fermented sweet rice and wheat. Rice wine is easy and cheap to make at home. Alcohol yeast cakes (酒麴, jiǔ qū) containing a combination of yeasts and molds can be found at Asian markets. For homemade rice wine recipes see Lia Andrews. *Medicinal Brewing; How to make wine out of honey, rice, and other grains.* (San Diego: Alcyone Press, 2014). or the recipe section of Lia Andrews. *7 Times a Woman; Ancient Wisdom on Health & Beauty for Every Stage of Your Life.* (San Diego: Alcyone Press, 2013).

Red Dragon (红龙, hónglóng) – A metaphor for menstruation in Inner Alchemy.

Shen (神, shén) – The spirit of the Heart and can also be translated as "consciousness." In TCM, the Heart houses the Mind. It also refers to the overarching spirit of the person. The Heart Shen is the part of a person that is conscious of being and integrates the other spirits of the four other spirits: the Hun, Po, Yi, and Zhi. Imbalance in the Heart causes the Shen to scatter, leading to mental and emotional disturbances.

Traditional Chinese Medicine (TCM) (中医, zhōngyī) – Often used to describe the standardized traditional medicine of China created by post-revolutionary China. It is also used to describe the broader traditional medicine that evolved in China and Taiwan. Some propose using a broader term such as Traditional Asian Medicine to include Japanese, Korean, and other evolutions of the medicine. TCM relies on acupuncture, moxibustion, qigong, herbal medicine, cupping, gua sha, and massage. In Asian countries is also includes bonesetting and chiropractic.

Wind (风, fēng) – Internally manifests as headaches, migratory pain, vertigo, seizures, or convulsions. Internal Wind is generated by a deficiency of Blood or Yin and/or an excess of Heat. External Wind refers to pathogenic invasion, as in bacterial and viral infections, which is accompanied by Heat or Cold. External Wind causes a superficial pulse. Internal Wind can cause a rigid and deviated tongue.

Women's Alchemy (女丹, nüdān) – Inner Alchemy specific to women. These include breast massage, ovarian massage, and jade egg practices. They traditionally focus on lessening or stopping menstrual flow and balancing women's reproductive organs for the purpose of spiritual advancement. In modern times they are often used for increasing health, vitality, and sensuality.

Yang (阳, yáng) – Relates to the insubstantial, Qi, the sun, heat, movement, excess, rising, morning, back side of the body.

Yang Deficiency (阳虚, yángxū) – Is a progression of Qi deficiency resulting in more weakness of function with the addition of Cold symptoms. Common signs include low back and knee weakness, soreness, and/or cold, loose stools early in the morning (cock's crow diarrhea), edema in the lower body, copious urination. urinary or fecal incontinence, and nocturia (night urination). Yang deficiency can affect the Spleen, Kidney, and Heart organ systems. It can be constitutional or caused by longstanding Qi Deficiency, Cold damage, physical overwork (includes excessive exercise), exhaustion. Yang deficiency presents as a pale tongue with wet coating and deep, slow pulse.

Yi (意, yì) – The spirit of the Spleen. It governs intellect, intention, and the ability to digest ideas and experiences. A weak Spleen and unbalanced digestion can cause fuzzy thinking, rumination, and impair cognition.

Yin (阴, yīn)– Relates to substantial, Blood and body fluids, the moon, cold, stillness, deficiency, sinking, evening, front side of the body.

Yin Deficiency (阴虚, yīnxū) – Is a progression of Blood deficiency resulting in more loss of substance with the addition of Heat symptoms. Common signs include dryness (dry cough, throat, skin, vagina), dizziness, constipation, poor memory, heat worse at night, night sweats, thirst, flushed cheeks, dark urine, 5 Hearts Heat (in the palms, feet, and head), insomnia, tinnitus, memory loss, excess libido, low back soreness, ache in the bones, and bright red menstrual blood. Yin deficiency can affect the Heart, Lungs, Stomach, and Kidneys. It can be constitutional or due to Heat or Fluid damage, chronic illness, excessive sexual activity, mental overwork, prolonged emotional distress, emotional trauma, or older age. Yin deficiency presents as a small red tongue, with scant or mirrored coating and a thin, rapid pulse.

Zhi (智, zhì) – The spirit of the Kidneys. It governs willpower and deepest purpose. If the Kidneys are weak there may be a lack of determination and follow through.

Zuo Yue Zi Water – literally "postpartum recovery water," is rice wine processed to remove the majority of the alcohol content. Dr. Shuqi Zhuang's brand is 廣和坐月子水 Guang He Zuo Yue Zi Shui – literally "Great Harmony Postpartum Recovery Water."

Resources

Nutrition

Pitchford, Paul. *Healing With Whole Foods; Oriental Traditions and Modern Nutrition.* (Berkeley: North Atlantic Books, 1993).

Ni, Maoshing. *Tao of Nutrition.* (Los Angeles: Tao of Wellness Press, 1987).

Fermentation

Andrews, Lia. *Medicinal Brewing; How to Make Wine Out of Honey, Rice, and Other Grains.* (San Diego: Alcyone Press, 2014).

Buhner, Stephen Harrod. *Sacred and Herbal Healing Beers: The Secrets of Ancient Fermentation.* (Brewers Publications, 1998).

Katz, Sandor. *Wild Fermentation: The Flavor, Nutrition, and Craft of Live-Culture Foods.* (Vermont: Chelsea Green Publishing Company, 2003).

Cultures for Health: www.culturesforhealth.com. Variety of ferments available for purchase including koji and kefir.

Connecting with Plants

Cowan, Eliot. *Plant Spirit Medicine: The Healing Power of Plants.* (Columbus: Swan Raven & Company, 1991).

Buhner, Stephen Harrod. *Sacred Plant Medicine: The Wisdom in Native American Herbalism.* (Rochester: Bear & Company, 1996).

Chinese Herbs

Chinese herbs can be purchased from licensed acupuncturists.

Wing Hop Fung: www.WingHopFung.com (Chinese herbs, teas, and dried foods)

Dragon Herbs: www.DragonHerbs.com (Chinese herbs, acupuncture products)

Chinese Ingredients

99 Ranch Market: www.99Ranch.com. Stores in California, Nevada, Washington, and Texas.

Mitsuwa Market (Japanese): www.mitsuwa.com/english/index.html. Stores in California, New Jersey and Chicago.

Nijiya Market (Japanese): www.nijiya.com. Stores in Californiia, New York, and Hawaii.

Fertility

For laypeople: Ni, Daoshing. *The Tao of Fertility: A Healing Chinese Medicine Program to Prepare Body, Mind, and Spirit for New Life.* (New York: Harper Collins Pulishers, 2008).

For acupuncturists: Lyttleton, Jane. *Treatment of Infertility with Chinese Medicine.* (China: Churchill Livingstone, 2004).

Postpartum Care

Jing Mommy: traditional Taiwanese postpartum services including frozen meals. English-speaking. Retail bottled Yue Zi Shui (postpartum water). www.JingMommy.com, 810 N. Nogales St. Walnut, CA 91789 Phone: 626-217-7539

Placenta Encapsulation

Placenta Benefits: www.PlacentaBenefits.info

Placenta Bakery: www.PlacentaBakery.com

Credits

Cover
Book Cover Illustrations:
www.backgrounds.mysitemyway.com, www.shutterstock.com
www.depositphotos.com; © ColorValley #11465725; © nataliia-ku #7038038
www.EvidenceoftheHand.com
Cover Design by Lia Andrews

Interior
Layout Design by Miya of PXP Design
Figure Illustrations by Lia Andrews

Index

U

V

W

Y

Z

About the Author

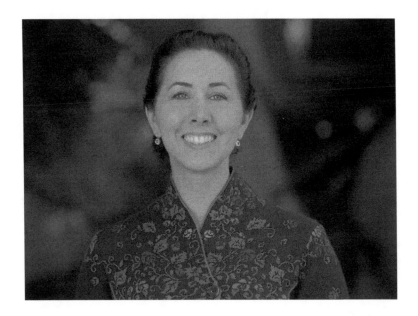

Dr. Lia G. Andrews, DAOM, L.Ac. was born in Norwalk, Connecticut. She attended Bryn Mawr College and the College of William & Mary, where she received her BA in International Studies. She received her Masters in Acupuncture and Traditional Chinese Medicine (MATCM) from Yo San University. Dr. Andrews received her Doctorate of Acupuncture and Oriental Medicine (DAOM) from Pacific College of Oriental Medicine. She is licensed nationally and in the state of California. Also in print is her doctoral capstone on traditional postpartum care: "Partial Translation of 'Postpartum Recovery Program; a Manual of Rules and Recipes for the Postpartum Woman.'" (DAOM capstone, Pacific College of Oriental Medicine, 2013).

Dr. Andrews has traveled to Brazil, Thailand, and China in her study for natural healing. She practices in the clinic she founded with her mother, Dr. Judith Andrews, Cinnabar Acupuncture Clinic & Spa in San Diego, California.

Also Available from Dr. Andrews

Health Awakening Series

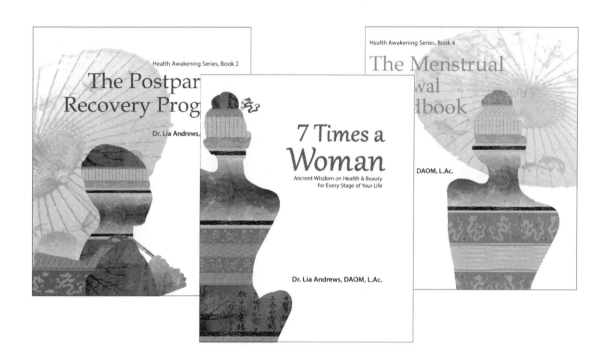

Book 1 - 7 Times a Woman
Book 2 - The Postpartum Recovery Program™

UPCOMING:
Book 3 - The Menstrual Renewal Handbook
Book 4 - Secrets of the Daoist Courtesan
Book 5 - Return to Spring (Menopause)
Book 6 - Detoxification
Book 7 - Empowerment

13371255R00144

Printed in Poland
by Amazon Fulfillment
Poland Sp. z o.o., Wrocław